# ACHIEVEMENTS IN RESIDENTIAL SERVICES FOR PERSONS WITH DISABILITIES

# ACHIEVEMENTS IN RESIDENTIAL SERVICES FOR PERSONS WITH DISABILITIES
## Toward Excellence

Edited by

**Tony Apolloni, Ph.D.**
California Institute on Human Services
Sonoma State University

**Joanna Cappuccilli, M.A.**
Human Services Associates
Santa Rosa

and

**Thomas P. Cooke, Ph.D.**
Department of Special Education
Sonoma State University

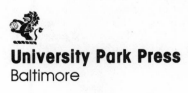

**University Park Press**
Baltimore

**UNIVERSITY PARK PRESS**
International Publishers in Science, Medicine, and Education
233 East Redwood Street
Baltimore, Maryland 21202

Typeset by University Park Press, Typesetting Division.
Manufactured in the United States of America by
The Maple Press Company.

Funded in part by the Instructional Television Consortium,
The California State University and Colleges, 1801 East Cotati
Avenue, Rohnert Park, California 94928.

**Library of Congress Cataloging in Publication Data**

Main entry under title:

Achievement in residential services for persons with
disabilities.

Proceedings of a conference held in Pomona, Calif.,
Dec. 14–15, 1977.
Includes index.
1. Developmentally disabled services—United States
—Congresses. 2. Community mental health services—
United States—Congresses. I. Apolloni, Tony.
II. Cappuccilli, Joanna. III. Cooke, Thomas P.
IV. Title: Toward excellence.
HV3006.A3A25      362.3'0973      79-22077
ISBN 0-8391-1541-5

# CONTENTS

# CONTRIBUTORS

**Tony Apolloni, Ph.D.**
California Institute on Human
  Services
Sonoma State University
1801 E. Cotati Avenue
Rohnert Park, California 94928

**Timothy C. Blackburn, Ph.D.**
Department of Special Education
University of the Pacific
Stockton, California 95211

**William Bronston, M.D.**
Department of Developmental
  Services
714 P Street
Sacramento, California 95404

**Joanna Cappuccilli, M.A.**
Human Services Associates
1639 Manzanita Avenue
Santa Rosa, California 95404

**Thomas P. Cooke, Ph.D.**
Department of Special Education
Sonoma State University
1801 E. Cotati Avenue
Rohnert Park, California 94928

**Wade Hitzing, Ph.D.**
Center for the Development of
  Community Alternative Service
  Systems
Medical Center, University
  of Omaha
Omaha, Nebraska 68131

**Mel Knowlton**
Office of Mental Retardation
Bureau of Community Programs
Health and Welfare Building,
  Room 302
Harrisburg, Pennsylvania 19120

**Charles A. Peck, M.A.**
Department of Education
Sonoma State University
1801 E. Cotati Avenue
Rohnert Park, California 94928

**Betty Pieper**
R.D. #1 Ridge Road
Scotia, New York 12302

**Gerald Provencal, M.S.W.**
Macomb-Oakland Regional Center
16200 19 Mile Road
Mt. Clemens, Michigan 48044

**G. Allan Roeher, Ph.D.**
Canadian Association for the
  Mentally Retarded
21 Colwick Drive
Willowdale, Ontario, Canada
  M2K G4

**Georgeanne White-Blackburn,
M.A.**
Developmental Assistance and
  Training Associates
13401 Sargent Avenue
Galt, California 95632

**Albert Zonca**
Sonoma County Citizen
  Advocacy, Inc.
853 Fourth Street
Santa Rosa, California 95402

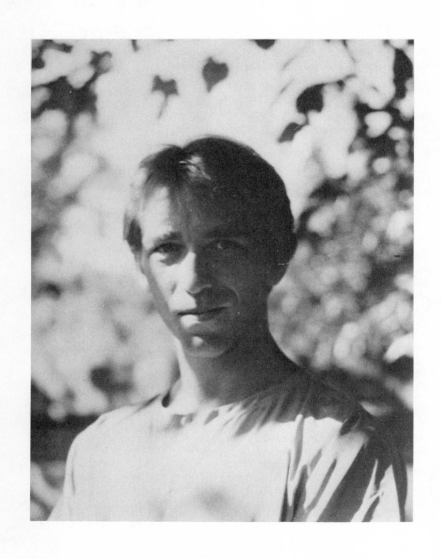

# PREFACE

This book offers a record of "Toward Excellence," a conference on residential services for persons with special developmental needs that occurred in Pomona, California, on December 14 and 15, 1977. This conference was conceptualized and presented to acquaint the leadership of California's residential services movement with "cutting edge" ideology and procedures. The speakers who shared so eloquently at the conference were contemporary heroes in a minority group struggle toward equal opportunity. In addition, the editors of this volume have seen fit to include material that, while not a direct component of the conference, seemed to add cogent contributions to the conference topic. Specifically, Al Zonca's chapter on advocacy; Cap Peck's, Georgeanne White-Blackburn's, and Tim Blackburn's empirical review of community living arrangements; and Joanna Cappuccilli's pictorial essay on Somerset Home School provide enrichment of the conference materials.

The presentations of "Toward Excellence" contained in this volume were prepared by men and women who are deeply committed to attacking social inequities faced by citizens with disabilities. William Bronston, Gerald Provencal, Wade Hitzing, Mel Knowlton, and Allan Roeher currently occupy leadership positions in major service systems. Betty Pieper, Joanna Cappuccilli, and Tony Apolloni share the practical concern of establishing a high quality living situation for an immediate family member. The writers share other binding characteristics. They have spent most of their professional careers promoting, designing, implementing, or managing community-based residential service systems for persons with special developmental needs. All are personally committed to the value of creating alternatives to institutions; all have experience in deinstitutionalization programs; most have been employees in state institutions, and have had extensive experience in developing staff training programs for human services workers. These pioneers were asked to alert the conference participants to innovative "real-world" alternatives to state institutions while identifying the major problems and opportunities in the process of instituting preferred futures for California citizens who are labeled "developmentally disabled."

William Bronston is Medical Director for the Developmental Services Department of the California Health and Welfare Agency. Bill is known by all as a man of unexcelled zeal. He heads statewide committees on staff training, interdepartmental coordination, creative and cultural affairs, and prevention. His contributions articulate rationale and strategy for creating and expanding alternatives to institutional models. He outlines several sets of concrete considerations for developing humane, normalizing alternatives to state institutions.

Gerald Provencal is the Acting Director of the Macomb-Oakland Regional Center in Michigan. He serves as a member of the Task Force on Residential Training and the Standing Committee on Adult Community Placement for the Michigan Department of Mental Health. Gerald has designed and organized deinstitutionalization plans (including 2,300 consumers at the Willowbrook Developmental Center), and has worked extensively with community care providers and parents. Mr. Provencal's presentation describes the Macomb-Oakland Regional Center program and reviews two residential alternatives (group homes and community training homes). Moreover, he supplies an overview of the staff training strategies intrinsic to his agency's system and shares its strengths and weaknesses, including some trade secrets on how this training program works. Finally, he makes a passionate plea for maintaining a sense of urgency and a sense of agency responsibility toward community-based service development.

Betty Pieper is a leading parent in the National Association for Retarded Citizens and the National Spina Bifida Association. She has written several publications on aspects of human services from a consumer's perspective. Her experience as a parent of a daughter who is disabled has provided her with a wealth of insight into system change, which she shares willingly and articulately. Joanna Cappuccilli is sister to an adolescent brother labeled "autistic." Joanna has a history of diligent service in a variety of human service positions, including experience as an assistant to Wolf Wolfensberger at Syracuse University. She currently serves as an instructor of developmentally disabled students at Santa Rosa Junior College and on numerous voluntary associations for the developmentally disabled. Ms. Pieper and Ms. Cappuccilli provide an overview of societal attitudes, legal considerations, and funding issues that are important for the development of exemplary, community-based service systems. They also review problems faced by consumers in their struggles to establish more integrated residential alternatives and outline futuristic principles to protect human rights and aid in normalizing human services.

In her Somerset Home School chapter Ms. Cappuccilli highlights the personalities and growth histories of six "severely, multiply handicapped" children who live in Somerset Home, a community care facility located in Sacramento, California. This program recently received recognition from the President's Commission on Mental Retardation for being judged one of the 20 most outstanding residential facilities in the United States. The chapter reviews the developmental histories and current needs of the children who live in Somerset Home and illustrates that even medically fragile children can be served in community-based programs. The chapter depicts a unique program for a group of youngsters typically considered to hold little possibility of community placement.

Wade Hitzing is Director of the Center for the Development of Community Alternative Service Systems and former Division Director for the Eastern Nebraska Community Office of Retardation. He has a long and productive history of publications, presentations, grant management, training, and consultation in the area of residential services staff development in Michigan and Nebraska. Dr. Hitzing provides an overview of the structure and functions of the Eastern Nebraska Community Office of Retardation (ENCOR) and summarizes a number of important lessons to be learned from ENCOR and from other advanced community service systems. These lessons relate to: 1) the relative importance of philosophy versus technology in achieving service advances, 2) some of the problems associated with permanent, facility-based continua, 3) the value of designing and delivering services on an individual basis, and 4) the crucial importance of developing the most integrated aspects of service systems before supplying specialized services.

Al Zonca is executive director of Sonoma County Citizen Advocacy, Inc., a nationally recognized multidimensional personal advocacy system that incorporates citizen, broker, parent, and self-advocacy components. He is a leader in the advocacy movement in California. Mr. Zonca's chapter on advocacy adds a critical element to a text on community living arrangements. His discussion of various forms of advocacy offers insight that leads us away from oversimplified notions of citizen advocacy. Although not a part of the original "Toward Excellence" conference, Mr. Zonca's chapter is critical to the topic.

Mel Knowlton is the Director for the Bureau of Community Programs, Office of Mental Retardation, Commonwealth of Pennsylvania. He formerly served as the Director of Residential Services for the Eastern Nebraska Community Office of Retardation and as director of an Association for Retarded Citizens. Mr. Knowlton has extensive experience as a consultant, lobbyist, and expert witness on issues related to developmental services. His publications include *An Apartment Living Plan to Promote Integration and Normalization of Mentally Retarded Adults* (1), of which he was a co-author. Mr. Knowlton's chapter outlines the exemplary, community-based service system that exists in Pennsylvania and charts the future directions for this large, long-established model. These directions include: 1) more emphasis on multiply handicapped, medically fragile consumers, 2) fewer group homes and more individualized modes of service, 3) increased consumer participation in planning and delivering services, 4) efforts to minimize worker "burn-out," and 5) expanded emphasis on developing consumers' ability to control their own destinies.

Charles A. Peck is a senior associate with Human Services Associates. He also works as a consultant to a number of other developmental services agencies, including the California State Department of Education and the California State Department of Developmental Services. Mr. Peck has been active in program development, applied research, and program evaluation efforts in educational, vocational, and residential settings. Georgeanne White-Blackburn is a consultant to the Governor's Office (California) and the State Department of Education. She is currently working with the Chancellor's Office of the California State University and Colleges on a special project aimed at integrating community volunteers into agencies serving exceptional people. Her publications and presentations range from vocational workshop production strategies to personalized systems of instruction. Dr. Timothy C. Blackburn was director of the Community Re-Entry Project at Stockton State Hospital for 3 years. During that time, he was responsible for the development, testing, and implementation of programs aimed at assisting individuals to successfully re-enter and remain in the community. Currently he is Assistant Professor of Special Education at the University of the Pacific. He also serves as a special consultant to the California State Department of Education. Together, Mr. Peck, Ms. White-Blackburn, and Dr. Blackburn review the research literature relative to community living arrangements. They summarize the achievements of research efforts to date, and note some of the factors that limit the generality of the findings. Finally, they describe how the concepts and goals of normalization may reshape research and program development efforts directed toward forging high quality community living arrangements.

Allan Roeher is Executive Vice President of the Canadian Association for the Mentally Retarded. He has published and lectured internationally and has served as an advisor to various countries, especially with regard to the training of developmental services personnel and on innovative approaches to program delivery. Dr. Roeher has guided the development of a nationwide series of complementary research and demonstration projects, which has included the development of five university-affiliated centers. His current activities include supervising the implementation of regional comprehensive community service projects throughout Canada in order to bridge gaps between knowledge and practice. Dr. Roeher reviews historical and contemporary considerations in Canada's efforts to establish community-based services for citizens labeled "mentally retarded." He places particular emphasis on the development of comprehensive manpower development models, and reviews the career ladder and related training systems that exist in Canada.

Tony Apolloni holds appointments as a special education faculty member at Sonoma State University and as a psychologist at Sonoma State Hospital. He has served as a consultant to numerous state and local agencies in the areas of residential services design, evaluation, curriculum development, and staff training. Dr. Apolloni has published widely on topics related to residential service staff training and is guardian of a mentally retarded sister who lives in a group home.

In the final chapter, Dr. Apolloni summarizes common elements in progressive service systems and outlines important challenges to establishing high quality residential alternatives. The challenges discussed by Dr. Apolloni include: 1) establishing service continua, 2) establishing networks of community support services, 3) counteracting the influences that inhibit deinstitutionalization, 4) actualizing the principles of normalization, 5) involving consumers in service development, 6) gaining broad-based public support, 7) adopting the developmental model, 8) engendering advocacy, 9) stimulating communication between the service-providing and scientific communities, and 10) fostering inter-departmental cooperation in government.

This volume was made possible by the cooperation of many people. The editors offer sincere thanks to Dr. Stuart Cooney, Director of the Instructional Television Consortium, for his many contributions. Gratitude is also expressed to California's Developmental Services Training Committee for supporting the production of this manuscript and the conference that it records. Finally, special thanks are extended to Rhonda Bellmer for her capable editorial assistance and to Jane Wilder, Margaret Saal, and Marsh Rose, who painstakingly prepared the various drafts of this document.

Thomas P. Cooke, Ph.D.

**REFERENCE**
1. Fritz, M., Wolfensberger, W., and Knowlton, M. 1971. An Apartment Living Plan to Promote Integration and Normalization of Mentally Retarded Adults. Canadian Association for the Mentally Retarded, Downsview, Ontario, Canada.

To Anita and Dean
based on the intention
that they may continue to live like other people

# ACHIEVEMENTS IN RESIDENTIAL SERVICES FOR PERSONS WITH DISABILITIES

# THE SHAPE
# OF A MARATHON

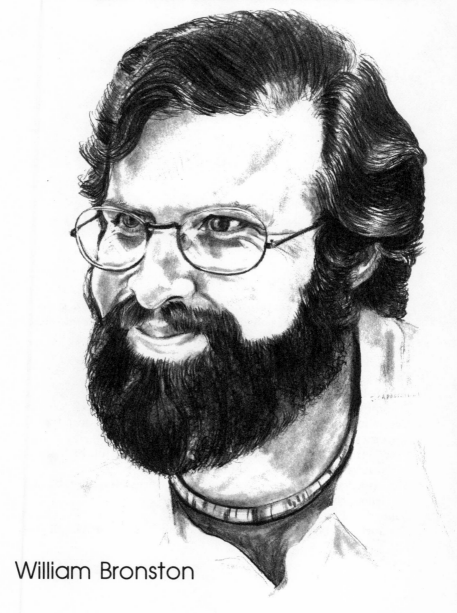

William Bronston

## NORMALIZATION

*There officially exists in California a philos-*ophy of services that is based deeply on values. It submits that in order to grow, each person deserves:

Love, honor, and freedom from stigma throughout life
Celebration of being special
A life-sharing family, home, and nurturing support
A community of concern and friendship
Economic security, health, and the full benefit of modern technology with a varied continuum of services
Freedom from the threat of injury due to pollution of food, air, water, and the earth on which we dwell
The opportunity to grow, learn, choose, work, rest, play, be nourished, to experience well-being
Solitude when needed
Comfort and beauty in which to discover himself or herself

The power to improve his or her environment
Justice
The dignity of risk, joy, and growth of spirit
A valid social future

Such philosophy sums up many of the deepest held beliefs about quality of life. These beliefs are at the root of our current and emerging civil rights and human services laws and standards.

How we, as human beings, are perceived decides how we are treated in society. Our judicial system declared its stand to defend the virtue and inalienable right for life: a commitment to change and growth, respect for each person based on individual identity, equality of opportunity, access to resources, full social integration, the right to privacy, the ability to exercise a voice in social affairs, and self-determination. These rights are rooted in and interpreted from our constitutional guarantees. They have been translated over recent years and summed up in the principle of normalization in human service. This principle forms a bridge between ideas expressed in our ideal cultural values and their implementation in society's caregiving structures. Normalization in theory and operation offers a standard of minimum acceptability on which human services must be conceived, planned, provided, and judged.

Normalization advocates the use of *means* that are culturally normative in order to offer a person life conditions *at least as good* as those of the average citizen and, as much as possible, to enhance and support personal behaviors, appearance, experience, status, and reputation to the greatest degree possible, at any given time, for each individual according to his or her special developmental needs (1, 2).

Normalization insists upon accentuating the positive and eliminating the negative by doing everything possible to integrate people who have special needs into everyday lives so that they may enjoy all we value for ourselves.

Normalization dictates use of the least restrictive or drastic means to help people grow and change to avoid stifling personal liberty. This notion also applies to how we socially burden or enhance human beings with our labels, the use of technology, the location and appearances of the buildings and spaces where services are carried on, and the image and impact of the kinds and numbers of service workers employed. All these influence how people served are seen and are decisive in shaping everyone's expectations, actions, and therefore the benefits or outcomes of service for individuals.

What is the best way to assist people in society to achieve and enjoy the fruits of that society? How do we assure not only that we do no harm, but that we uplift the persons we serve in the eyes of their fellow citizens? How do we balance the clinical or educational benefit of using methods that improve competence and performance with the cost in status and reputation of culturally stigmatizing measures? How do we protect the sense of personal well-being, confidence, dignity, and pride of a person in an interdependent relation with services and staffs who do not, or will not, identify with that person as a peer of equal worth? How do we recognize the right to treatment and help that each person possesses in our society, while eliminating ineffective programs that represent deprivations of liberty and impose overly restrictive alternatives? How do we implement the responsibility as teachers and caregivers such that, in the words of John Donne, "No man is an island, entire of itself; every man is a piece of the continent, a part of the main . . . any man's death diminishes me, because I am involved in mankind . . ."?

This anthology is already a history book, yet the experience and values addressed here are almost nonexistent in the literature of developmental services.

This summing up of the state of the art in the creation of lifestyle services paints a picture of what has happened in several places. It is up to us to garner the lessons of this search for excellence, and push forward to an even more civilized and humane future. Presented here is the tapestry of ideas and practice, woven together, one giving impetus to another in a progressive act of improvement.

Clearly, Nebraska with its ENCOR experience became the cornerstone for the fundamental challenge to North American human services. The uncompromising commitment to an ideology of service, developed in great detail as the principle of normalization, made almost everything that preceded it in the field obsolete. There is no way to fully measure the impact of such a contribution. It exploded the possible in the field through an idea, heroic leaders, and a concrete model. The idea, like dandelion seed carried on the wind, spread to consumers, planners, teachers, service providers, advocates, and researchers alike. If we do our job well, we may at least derive the following service benefits or actions:

Institution placements prevented
Persons returned from institutions
Emotional breakdowns prevented
Family breakup averted
Loneliness dispelled
Health preserved or restored
Services or social participation enhanced
Proper treatment provided
Persons habilitated
Dollars saved
Personnel needs reduced
Justice rendered or preserved

We are still in the first mile, a mere decade, into a marathon that will stretch on and on toward the excellence of attainment and fulfillment. We can draw ourselves forward together into this demanding run. Tangible rewards of the race are reaped while we labor with both love and science to transform our society. Intangible intimate rewards of the effort are realized as personal records that are continually broken every minute of the way toward our common destiny.

It is in this spirit that this material is set forth. It is intended to create understanding of the continuum of appropriate help and living arrangement services needed for people with special developmental needs. It is meant to be a small commitment to common humanity and respect for every human being.

## REFERENCES

1. Wolfensberger, W. 1972. The Principle of Normalization in Human Services. National Institute on Mental Retardation, Toronto.
2. *Way to Go*. 1978. University Park Press, Baltimore.

# MATTERS OF DESIGN

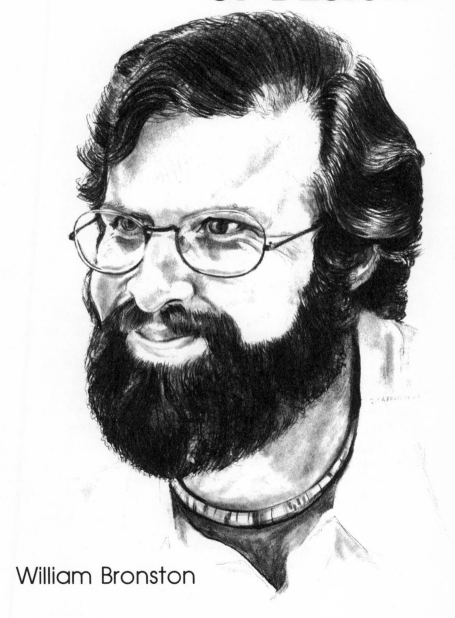

William Bronston

## THE SUBSTANCE OF THE LIVING ARRANGEMENT ISSUE

*In the chapters ahead, there are sequences of* basic ideas, principles, and models that summarize the key contemporary living arrangement issues. The following outlines offer some key checklists that provide a reference and priority for the most important issues. Recognizing the power of environment in our culture to act as a medium of status and identity, we must take stock of the attitudes and philosophies that underlie the design of a residence. We must ask and honestly answer:

1. What is the meaning embodied in or conveyed by the environment?
2. For whose convenience was the environment designed?
3. What role expectancies does the environmental design impose upon the clients-users?

We rely almost entirely on the assumption that people with special needs do not have equality or common value as people and, once alienated from their families, require *paid for* care. Our system is based on buying help—professional services, shift staff. Buying help is an industry that we manipulate—parent and public official alike. Our cultural institutions have not, as many European and non-Anglo societies have, embraced our vulnerable members as part of the family of man, deserving love, comfort, dignity, and intimate relations. Thus, we labor to create a situation whose foundation is always dangerously weak and subject to the winds of cruelty and inhumanity that have blown strongly in our century.

Stereotypes predominate. We must find ways to eliminate popular beliefs, which are based upon what the public has learned from the past about disability. We must teach our citizens to believe in our capacity to emancipate people with disabilities through new environments and magnificent scientific achievements.

Having been pushed to the margins of society, looking and acting very differently, congregated, and subjected to benign hopelessness, our constituency has been devastated in the eyes of most people. We seem to be discovering truths about life and growth that are old hat for valued sectors of society, but are breakthroughs that must be fought for when people are labeled "retarded" or "disabled" in one form or another.

This "discovery" of common sense, this celebration of the obvious in the design of decent living should evoke considerable embarrassment and even humble apology from the professions and bureaucracies that have teamed up to cling to institutions and service segregation.

## TRADITIONAL LIVING ARRANGEMENTS NETWORK

The traditional continuum of living arrangements has emphasized a network of facilities that includes:

Large state hospitals
Skilled nursing facilities
Intermediate care facilities
Residential school facilities
Board and care facilities          Ranging from small to large
Group home facilities

Semi-independent living situations

Independent living situations

} In one's own home, an apartment, a foster care situation, or a small family living group

Underlying this network, improperly identified as a continuum, has been the assumption that, the more complex and severe the individual's need and areas of dependency, the more likely it is that the person will be served in a large, segregated program. On the other hand, the assumption goes, the more competent and able the individual, the more likely it is that he or she will best live in a small home. A related assumption is that services (care and supervision) in large facilities where individuals are congregated (state hospitals, skilled nursing facilities) will be provided by staff who live away from the facility and work on a shift basis within it. Conversely, similar services in small, home-like facilities will be provided by "live-in" staff. Experience shows that these rigidly held assumptions are clearly outmoded. A need exists to reform this traditional outlook, whose continued existence is challenged by our evolving social values and technology.

When existing living arrangements are assessed against the principles and standards of normalization and civil rights guarantees, the following problems emerge:

1. Residential services are inflexible, built as they are on ponderous laws and regulations. Such services are *not* designed to assure movement through the system in keeping with an individual's growth. There is no *planned and assured option for physical movement* from program to program, or facility to facility, or for programmatic change within any given setting in accordance with individual needs, much less to provide for choices and transition.

2. There has not been a commitment to systematic programming in every living arrangement that supports and enhances individual growth and development and is intentional and universal.

3. There has not been a commitment to systematic staff development that would assure the availability of sufficient knowledgeable and competent service workers (including caregivers) fully grounded in program philosophy and progressively advancing toward career objectives with state sanction.

4. Program and facilities have not been designed according to a clear-cut continuum of less restrictive alternatives to individual liberty and autonomy.
5. Living arrangements have not been designed to be appropriate to the chronological age of the individual. Too frequently there has been a mixing of individuals of widely disparate ages, outside of natural, foster, or adoptive family situations. This has led to poor personal images and low program expectations for both children and adults alike.
6. Individuals with different categorical labels and types of disability have been mixed in the same facility. This has resulted in a devalued image and program hodgepodge for the individuals involved, instead of providing them with opportunities and models for social integration with typical peers.
7. Current individual living arrangements have been maintained in spite of the fact that they are not the least restrictive alternative and where, as a result, the developmental needs of persons have not been met.
8. In the overwhelming majority of states, nowhere is there a complete continuum of living arrangements. Many individuals are placed according to what is locally available or in a more appropriate program far from home communities, rather than according to what is needed and desirable.
9. There is no statutory mandate for direct provision of living arrangements that meshes public and private resources appropriately, and that acts to eliminate the reality of excessive competition, duplication, and fragmentation.

## THE DESIGN FOR A TRANSITIONAL LIVING ARRANGEMENTS CONTINUUM

Because of the shortcomings identified of the traditional network of living arrangements, we can propose to remedy the situation with the design shown in Figure 1, a design that reduces pseudo-diversity to the most basic elements. Such a model acknowledges what exists and the need to strengthen and reinforce the preferred parts while providing disincentives for the unacceptable and undesirable components.

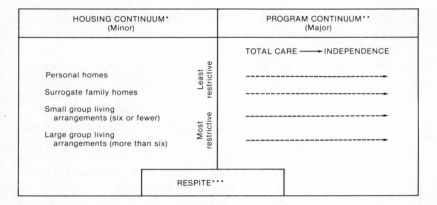

**Figure 1.** A transitional living arrangement continuum. *Includes facilities operating under both public and private auspices and those that are not for profit as well as those that are proprietary. **Clients in the housing (minor) continuum will be situated in the program (major) continuum according to their individual special developmental needs and program plan. ***Cuts across the living arrangements continuum, i.e., has both program and housing components.

## RATIONALE FOR THE DESIGN OF THE COMPREHENSIVE LIVING ARRANGEMENTS CONTINUUM

The housing continuum contains within it a full range of components from the ideal (least restrictive-most typical) to the least acceptable alternative to that ideal (most restrictive-least typical). It is assumed that any given individual with developmental services needs will come into the housing continuum at any point and, barring unforeseen circumstances, move along it progressively toward the ideal.

The program continuum likewise contains within it a full range of components from its beginning point—total care—to its goal— independence. It is assumed that any given individual will come into the continuum at any point and, again barring unforeseen circumstances, move progressively along it toward maximum autonomy and well-being.

Although the major and minor continua may be considered independently, they are interrelated components of the comprehensive living arrangements continuum. In this comprehensive continuum model, both program and housing needs must be addressed systematically and simultaneously.

Available experience in the nation establishes that there are all kinds of people with all kinds of problems in all kinds of settings getting all kinds of services. Thus, at any point on the program continuum—and, conversely, at given points in the program continuum—individuals can make their home at any point on the housing continuum.

Beyond these basics, a person's age is one of the most sensitive considerations that must be superimposed upon the major and minor continua. Separation by age, although basic to the respectful acknowledgment of a person and means by which to assure proper attitudes and program design, cannot be dogmatically exercised. A few considerations are central.

A person usually lives with parents or parent surrogates during childhood. Upon reaching the age of independence, individuals typically seek their own domicile. It is unusual in our culture for a person to return to or stay in his or her parents' home except for respite periods of transition, sanctuary, or the like.

Furthermore, it is only in the natural family that a range of age from infancy through adulthood is typical. Adults or teenagers near adulthood must be accorded an age status and culturally enhancing environment that does not further burden the image of "eternal child."

In relation to the issue of appropriate and enhancing living arrangements for children, if the maxim "support, do not supplant the family" cannot be achieved, then out-of-home placement for children must emphasize the most individualized of all relations. The younger the person, the more in need is that person of a single caregiver and continuity of care. Single-person living arrangements for children are preferred, coupled with social integration with typical peers in all activities.

Some examples of desirable service universals that are particularly relevant to living arrangements include:

1. Ready access
2 . Aesthetics of facility
3. Physically comfortable facility
4. Age-appropriate facilities and service approaches
5. Positive value image of service and clients
6. Intense programming
7. Individualization
8. Respectful, warm social interactions

9. Social integration
10. Meaningful participation of consumers and public
11. Self-renewal orientation
12. Receptivity to research
13. Ties to academia

The following considerations should help us to rank order alternatives on a *continuum:*

1. Support, not supplant, the natural home.
2. Use foster placement or family-like settings, especially for children.
3. If you must use a non-family setting, lease, don't buy.
4. Buy an existing structure, don't build.
5. Build a typical home, not special.
6. Build a special structure within the community, not isolated.

There seems to be at least four major arguments favoring small residential settings: 1) the group and residence do not attract undue attention by being larger than a large family; 2) the larger a grouping of perceived deviant individuals, the less likely it is that the neighborhood and its resources will absorb them; 3) large groups become self-sufficient, orient inward, and resist outward integration; and 4) when groups are larger than six or eight, house parents or resident advisors can no longer properly relate to individual group members and structure the group.

The setting in which persons are served should absolutely not be equated with the degree or complexity of their disability. Traditionally, our field has established the formula of placing the most disabled person in the most medical/segregated/congregate setting and considering normative dwellings only for independent or semi-independent living. In fact, the key and decisive variable is the competence and quality of the caregiver. That is to say, program is what counts. Thus, almost without exception, apartment dwellings could suffice for all our service needs, except where gross acute medical/hospital services were needed to stabilize a person for short-term duration. Benefits of apartment living are:

1. Flexibility in programming
2. Normalization for tenants
3. Integration of tenants into the community
4. Improvement of the cost-benefit ratio
5. Extension of the continuum of residential services

6. Quick start-up of program
7. Elimination of most or all zoning and building code barriers

Once we have exhausted less restrictive alternatives and are definitely faced with an out-of-home placement, 10 considerations must be simultaneously addressed. Our aim is to make possible a quality of life that matches as closely as possible family familiarity and security. Community living arrangements must be:

1. Normalizing and adaptive
2. Dispersed across and within population centers
3. Socially and physically integrated in the community
4. Age appropriate in setting design, decor, structures, and rhythms
5. Separate from other daily living functions, such as school, work, play
6. Small (size of group)
7. The least restrictive alternative setting and structure
8. Designed for high diversity of models (specialization)
9. In a continuum with other residential and nonresidential services
10. Supportive of staff-tenant relationships

The matter of staff-tenant relations seems the most delicate. The distance created by a professional (paid) caregiver as opposed to a person who seeks the caregiver relation based first on spontaneous friendship or love requires constant attention. The staff is a vital component in maximizing culturally typical relations, or "life sharing." Regardless, all living arrangements should maximize:

1. Diminishing rather than accentuating distinctions between staff and clients
2. Staff and clients sharing space, toilets, meals, real recreation, fun, vacations, joy, song, suffering, worship, etc.
3. Living with (not just close to) clients
4. Maximizing peer modeling
5. Enhancing direct contact by volunteers.

At a more system-wide level, such comprehensive and rational living arrangements models must be planned and generated by significant administrative commitment and structures. Such requirements include at least:

1. Community living branch in state government
2. Local community living arrangements provider agency
3. Performance agreements between local agencies and state government
4. Use of existing geopolitical boundaries for regional service areas
5. Mandatory and continuous personnel development and training
6. Evaluation and data collection capacity
7. Quarterly advance funding for start-up
8. Quality review mechanism and standards
9. Advocacy and monitoring safeguards
10. Development of normalized zoning and building codes and licensing rules (anti-ghettoization)

At the local/regional level of service delivery, a publicly funded and administered agency (quasi-public or public authority or joint powers board) is essential if state services (institutions) are to be decentralized and transformed. Only in this way can assurances be made to free parent organizations from clinging to archaic property and buildings and ultimately to become free of the role of provider of last resort.

This local/regional public agency must be responsible to:

1. Administer programs
2. Provide residential planning and services for all persons from the service area, including persons from the locale presently living in state institutions
3. Mobilize public support for residential services
4. Provide or purchase needed services to include: family subsidy, in-home support, foster placements, respite, crisis assistance, subsidized adoptive programs, independent living, semi-independent living, group living for six or fewer, specialized living programs
5. Develop local resources to support residents in nondomiciliary life needs

## FINALE: THE STARTING PLACE

Normal living settings represent only the structural hub if services are to be relevant, personal, and developmental. A number of satellite forces and conditions must keep the constellation in dynamic balance, depicted in Figure 2.

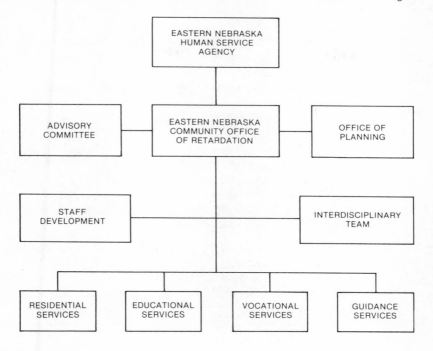

**Figure 2.** Constellation of essential service forces in a full continuum.

Institutions, however archaic, remain. As long as institutional models exist, every realistic effort must be made to upgrade their services and enhance the quality of life for those persons who reside and work there. Nevertheless, commitment must be made to stop all proposed institutional and residential construction, to eliminate plans for new traditional institutions, and to effect orderly deinstitutionalization with strict safeguards, advocacy, and monitoring.

In summary, four levels of action are called for: 1) increase community services and decrease need for residential places; 2) replace large institutions with small, dispersed, specialized residences and apartments; 3) return institution residents to society, community, or family; and 4) improve institutions as long as needed. These checklists but scratch the surface, yet the scope and possibilities of the situation are suggested. As each contributor to this volume describes his or her work, these criteria will correlate and take on concrete implications and interpretations.

# THE MACOMB-OAKLAND REGIONAL CENTER

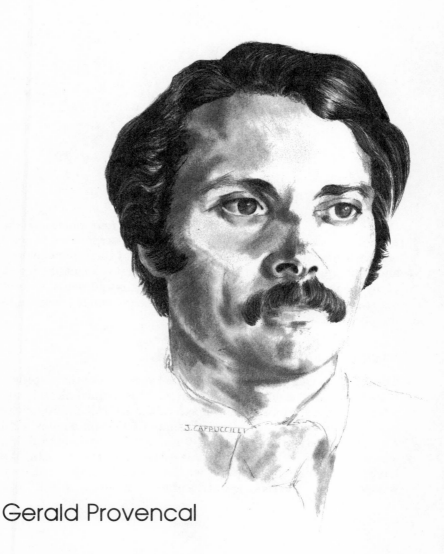

J. CAPPUCCILLI

Gerald Provencal

*This* *chapter* *focuses* *on* *four* *areas:* *1)* *the* agency I work for, 2) two of our residential alternatives, which I believe are unique, at least in some aspects of their management and staff training, 3) the training strategy that is an intrinsic part of my agency's programs, and 4) the strengths and weaknesses of our training per se, including some trade secrets on how our training program works.

## MACOMB-OAKLAND REGIONAL CENTER

The Macomb-Oakland Regional Center is one part of the state system of mental retardation services in Michigan. Macomb and Oakland counties are located just north of the Detroit metropolitan area. Their combined areas include some 1,300 square miles, with a total population of just under 2 million. We have high living standards in some spots and some strong poverty pockets. We have very educated people and we have people who are not very well educated. It is representative of most suburban areas.

Macomb-Oakland Regional Center is a state institution. By statute, we are responsible for every "mentally retarded" citizen who might need institutional services in our two-county area. This means that we have to admit people, discharge people, and maintain active legal responsibility for the care, training, and habilitation of over 800 clients in our two counties as well as a potential client caseload of over 35,000 individuals.

A brief history of our agency should give the reader a better perspective from which to judge the programs that I describe later in this chapter. The Macomb-Oakland Regional Center really began in 1971, in the minds of some parents and legislators. At that time, if you were "mentally retarded" and lived in Macomb or Oakland counties, you either stayed at home or went off to a state institution that was over 50 miles away. It was seen as a very positive step, in 1971, to build an institution that was both close to home and more individually accommodating than institutions of the past. Parents and legislators came together and talked with architectural firms and program consultants about what a good institution should look like. They discussed architectural design, program elements that should be in place, and the attributes of staff that should be recruited in order to build a "good institution." An architectural firm was hired to prepare the plans and the parents, legislators, and professionals in the area were very pleased with the 750-bed facility that was designed.

The Macomb-Oakland Regional Center was established by state statute in 1972. The people hired at that time, including myself, thought it a positive thing that we were going to have a better institution, but that it would be an even better thing if we didn't have any institution at all. We assembled a like-minded, core group of people who strongly believed that the best institution is not necessarily the best solution, and set out to make the institution obsolete before it opened.

We were in a very fortunate position at that time in that we were recognized as having a responsibility for citizens from our area who had previously gone to state institutions. As a result, we could go to any of the out-of-state institutions and ask for names and descriptive information of all residents who were native to our two-county area. This was very important to our placement efforts because our staff began to become familiar with, and identify with, individuals whom we felt could lead fuller lives in the larger community.

The institution staffs we worked with were skeptical about our objectives and they really didn't expect that we would move many people to the larger community. They didn't anticipate that we would be able to affect their overall operation greatly, and so they cooperated, without faith perhaps, but they cooperated.

The results of our efforts are noteworthy. There were 1,400 people from our catchment area living in state institutions in 1972. Today there are 600. We have moved 800 out! Over the last 5½ years, we have had 18 admissions to institutions, and over the last 2 years, we have had two. The institution that was originally planned for 750 people has 90 beds. During the period from 1972 until today, we have developed a wide range of housing alternatives to the institutions. We didn't quite meet our goal of making the "good institution" literally obsolete, but we are now sure that we never needed it. Although they don't all believe it, most parents and legislators also now realize that we didn't have to have the institution.

## COMMUNITY-BASED RESIDENTIAL ALTERNATIVES

Many times retarded citizens are placed in institutions almost by dafault. The consensus of opinion frequently is that, "The institution is the only place we can turn to." This rationale stems in part from the perception that if the natural parents of a "mentally retarded" citizen cannot maintain him or her at home, then no one else can either. If there are no relatives who can take on the responsibility from the parents, then the institution is sought as the last, if not the only, alternative.

Over the years, the absence of alternatives to the natural home and the institution has become so predictable that parents and professionals have stopped looking for them. With this search being either abbreviated or nonexistent, the institution takes on greater value as the alternative of choice; it appears to be the best alternative, even a good or desirable one. Institutional admission then completes a circle that owes much of its origin to self-fulfilling prophecy.

At Macomb-Oakland, we made a different use of the self-fulfilling prophecy. We discarded the notion that the institution ever had to be the "only thing left to turn to." We set out on a course to provide alternatives to parents of "mentally retarded" citizens who were unable to care for their sons and daughters at home; we essentially acted on the premise that, if we worked diligently at establishing preferable alternatives to the institution, we could eliminate all default admissions and move people to the larger community who were already inappropriately placed within institutions. This premise is rather simplistic, but we were convinced that the nature of the problem had been given too much credit for complexity.

## Group Homes

We have basically used two residential models in our efforts to make the institution unnecessary—the group home and the community training home. Our 30 group homes, none of which existed when we opened in 1972, range in size from 4 to 12 clients, the average being 7. We have about 250 people living in group homes. The average cost of the homes is approximately $35 per day per resident, made up by Supplemental Security Income payments, state monies, and Title XX match money. All of the group homes that we have are operated by nonprofit corporations. We run none of them directly. We contract for services. None of the 15 nonprofit corporations that now run our homes existed before fall, 1972. We began by working with people we thought might be interested in running group homes. We showed them how to incorporate and how to set up the kinds of alternative structures that we wanted.

The administrators or managers, who are primarily responsible for the homes, are usually college graduates with a cause. They generally are not too much concerned with making money; they want to do something for people.

The responsibilities of group home administrators are several. In addition to managing their home, their budget, and routine responsibilities for food, transportation, and so forth, they must also attend training sessions on a monthly basis and staff meetings on all their clients' individualized program plans on a quarterly basis.

Some of our homes are staffed by couples, but most are staffed by single people without live-in personnel. The average wage of direct care personnel is about $3.25 an hour. All the residents in our homes go to public school programs or to some other major community activity during the day. Habilitation programs also occur within the homes. The staffs that operate the homes are recruited by the people we contract with, in cooperation with us.

We do reserve a kind of veto power. If we know an individual is being hired and we don't think he or she has the proper qualifications, we insist that another person be selected. We have also demanded that some staff members be fired for a variety of reasons. Most of the staff members that are hired for group homes are college students.

Direct care staffs are recruited in several ways. One of the best has been going to colleges, universities, and community colleges, and talking to classes of students who are enrolled in human services curricula. Holding 3-day seminars has also been very helpful. We discuss the needs of "handicapped" people, talk about how human services have evolved, and discuss career opportunities for people interested in the field. These seminars have proved very effective in stimulating people to ask, "I might be interested in working in some capacity; could I sit down and talk about it further?"

The staff members living or working in our group homes are responsible for typical things: room, board, and supervision. They also have responsibility for some in-house programming. Every client living in one of our group homes receives in-house programming 5 days a week, which complements whatever is going on in their major activity outside of the home. For example, someone in a school program might receive speech and language instruction and also receive related instruction at home. In this example, the speech teacher would meet with group home staff and discuss ways of carrying the speech program over into the home.

## Community Training Homes

Our second major option to institutionalization is what we call the "community training home." The community training home concept is really an embellishment on the old foster home model. Foster parents are well known to human services. Usually, they are people who want to do something good for somebody. Traditionally, potential foster parents seek out an agency that has a clientele that can use their help. In other words, the foster parents initiate the relationship and the agency plays an almost passive selection role. We have taken a much different approach to the recruitment of foster parents and to the kinds of contributions they offer. We have a very aggressive recruitment program. We use classified advertisements, posters, and speaking engagements throughout our two-county area. We talk to natural parents, to existing foster parents, and to potential adoptive parents in hopes of generating interest in our community training program. We try to sell them on the challenges of living and working with a person who has special needs.

At the present time, we have 145 community training homes. The sizes of the homes range from one to three clients. The number is determined by the physical size of the house and by the management capability of the foster family. The cost of community training homes is about $25 a day per client, with the costs paid from Supplemental Security Income, state monies, and Title XX funds. About 95% of all the people living in our community training homes are children. Generally speaking, the group home program serves adults and the community training home program serves children; however, we are individualized in our approach to this so there are some variations. About 60% of the people living in group homes and community training homes have severe to profound mental retardation, and about 70% of these have serious secondary handicaps that, in the past, would have excluded them from community living.

We contract with all community training home foster parents and group home administrators by a written agreement that clarifies mutual expectations. Service providers must agree to supply room, board, supervision, and in-house programming 2 hours a day. Further responsibilities of the community training home operator are attendance at monthly training meetings, completion of monthly reports, meeting with each client's social worker on a monthly basis, and attendance at quarterly staff meetings. They must also satisfy things that are part of routine community life like taking people to doctor appointments, on shopping trips, and so forth.

The qualifications for operating a community training home are based upon both objective and interpretive criteria. The objective standards are building requirements, such as 90 square feet of bedroom space for each individual in the home, and placement standards, such as a maximum of three clients in the same home and a total maximum of seven people per home, including foster children and the members of the natural family.

The interpretive kinds of qualifications are probably the most important and the most difficult to evaluate. We talk in depth to potential candidates about expectations. We want to know just what would be anticipated of a new member of their household.

Would there be high expectations or would the new resident be perceived as being too helpless for it to matter? Does the candidate really want to make the client a part of the family or plan to treat the client in a passive way? We want to know what kinds of disciplinary methods are used in the home. We want to see if spanking or abusive language is used. We think that it is important whether or not potential foster parents are consistent in handling their own children and their own affairs. We are interested in whether or not the family thinks that the client coming into their home can make a contribution to the entire dynamic of the household or if he or she will just be an observer. We want to make certain that they see the person with special needs as a part of the family, and as an active participant within it. We seek candidates who view our client as somebody they want to accept fully and who are not interested primarily either in money or in working their way into heaven.

With regard to staff recruitment, the group home program is self-sustaining. Once we begin to do business with vendors, they take on the task of recruitment. They attract college students through informational meetings as described, advertise in the classified section of newspapers, follow up on interest shown by institutional staff looking for new challenges, and essentially take advantage of all known methods of stimulating interest in their programs among potential employees.

On the other hand, we are exclusively responsible for the recruitment of all foster parents for community training homes. We make use of several techniques. Some of the most successful are classified advertisements in local papers, adoption agency referrals and solicitations, public service announcements on both radio and television, and bulletins and posters distributed to schools, libraries, and community centers. We have had success in following through on the referrals of other foster parents, and even natural parents. As a result of these initiatives, we receive between 30 and 50 inquiries each month. Of these 30–50, only 1 or 2 eventually become foster parents. There are a vast number of reasons for applicants failing to complete the process required for foster parenting. Often, we feel people have not applied for the right reasons; they could not and will not be as considerate as they should be, or the time demands of being a service provider are too great. Others are not willing to complete our reports, to attend staff meetings, and so on. We want to have a program that provides an alternative for people that is far superior to an institution. To achieve this, we must place high expectations and high demands on the people who operate our community training homes. We strive to attract a large group of applicants so that we can be highly particular when selecting foster parents.

## TRAINING RESIDENTIAL SERVICES PERSONNEL

### Training Responsibilities

Our experience at Macomb-Oakland Regional Center has been instructive regarding the ways training can fit into the overall deinstitutionalization process. In 1972, many staff members and I felt that one way to get alternatives to institutions off the ground was to do a better job at recruiting and training staff and making better use of the existing foster home and group home concepts. It had been my experience that most foster parents approach the agency. Agencies do not approach them. The same is true for group home administrators. It also has been my experience that many of the best potential foster parents and group administrators are never even aware that such programs exist, or if they are aware, they perceive them as being ventures that only the elderly, very kind of heart, extremely patient, or other very exceptional people are interested in doing. We wanted to change this perception and we wanted to take advantage of the skills of people who could offer much but were unlikely to make the first contact. So we mounted an aggressive recruitment and training campaign aimed at this population. The results have been very worthwhile.

We now have several hundred foster parents, adoptive parents, natural parents, and group home staffs living and working with highly difficult clients in the sense that most of them function at levels of severe to profound retardation and have significant secondary handicaps. We have been able to return these clients to home communities because we have selected the right people to receive them and we have taken very seriously our responsibility to ready the receivers. We select foster parents and group home personnel who are not only well qualified and interested in working with people who have special needs, but who are also committed to learning themselves. In this regard, we have found that the desire to *increase* knowledge of theories, trends, and techniques is a far better indicator of foster parent effectiveness than years as a parent, educational degree, or years of background in the field. The importance of receptivity to new knowledge and directions from the agency cannot be oversold as a critical factor in community placement success. As a matter of fact, our experience has led us to believe that if we carefully select and prepare the people who will be receiving the person leaving the institution, virtually anyone can move to the community at large. This belief has led us to place tremendous efforts in training foster parents and group home personnel.

In relation to the points on selection and preparation, it has also been our experience that there is no prerequisite skill or ability that a client must acquire to ensure adequate placement adjustment. There is more than a bit of irony in this discovery—many dedicated professionals are still looking for predictive characteristics for community placement success within the personality makeup or adaptive behavior profile of their clients. Many dedicated professionals are still trying to sort out the high risk people from the low risk people. Unfortunately, they are characterizing people rather than situations as risky. This notion has to change.

Institutions spend a great deal of time training attendants. One must have approximately 240 hours of inservice training on a variety of topics to work directly with the "retarded" who live in Michigan institutions, for example. Yet we all know that the wards serving institutionalized clients are understaffed and that attendants hardly ever have a chance to use the skills they learn within inservice classes. Relatively little money has been appropriated, or imagination spent, on the other hand, on training people who are taking clients out of institutions. It's no wonder that clients are returning to institutions from the community.

We can develop all the residential alternatives we want, but if people keep bouncing back into institutions because the folks out there are not ready for them, we haven't done very much. The National Association of Superintendents of Public Residential Facilities regularly publishes statistics on where institutions are going. Their data show that over 50% of people returning to institutions after trying to make it in the community return because they "fail to adjust." Nowhere is there any mention that they have been let down by an unambitious social worker or by an untrained foster parent who "failed to adjust." We in the field have a responsibility to provide environments wherein individual clients can adjust. Clients have no obligation to adjust; we have an obligation to assure adjustment. I cannot overstress this point; it's too critical.

## Curriculum Content

We decided that training was going to be an elementary part of our program. We didn't have any educators on the staff, nor did we have any members who really even knew much about training. We just had people who felt that it was important to train foster parents and group home personnel. So we assembled a large group of people who were knowledgeable about education. We found them by writing letters explaining our interests to community colleges, universities, University Affiliated Facilities, mental health departments, and departments of social services. We asked representatives from these agencies to meet with us to help identify a training strategy. Thirty people were interested enough to attend our meeting. Everybody liked the idea, but no one wanted to consider funding. Everybody endorsed the need, but nobody wanted to write the curriculum. Everybody thought it was a terrific idea, the greatest since sliced bread, but no one wanted to do the work. Nobody wanted to go to night meetings. Nobody wanted to send out brochures, and nobody wanted to help assemble the topics for potential training objectives. And so we saw another reason why no one is ever trained. Nobody wanted to do it because it wasn't anybody's job.

Eventually, two other people and I decided to put our efforts where our mouths were and prepare a curriculum. We didn't proceed in any terribly scholarly fashion to find out what topics should be included in the curriculum. Instead, we sent out a well-thought-out questionnaire to all the foster parents in our community to see what they thought should be included. We asked them just two questions: what personal skills would make your job easier and what personal skills would make life better for the person living in your home? That's all, two things. Not 100 questions, not 16 questions, we didn't do a factor analysis, we just asked two questions. What would make your job better for you and what would make it better for the client you serve?

We received an extensive list of items which we proceeded to melt down to 50 potential topic areas (see Table 1). The topics included the role of group homes, first aid procedures, seizure information, the use of volunteers, insurance, discharge policies, advocacy, and toilet training. We took the 50 topics and divided them into two categories: mandatory core topics that we determined everyone must be exposed to, and an elective group of topics that we felt were important but not as fundamentally so as the first group. The core topics include orientations on: 1) mental

**Table 1.**   Possible training and educational topics

☐ Role of Group Home
☐ Assisting Services
☐ Individual Programming
☐ Legal Considerations/Liability
☐ Orientation to Mental
 Retardataion
☐ First Aid
☐ Parent Involvement
☐ Menus/Diet/Nutrition
☐ Sexuality
☐ Neighborhood Relations
☐ Record Keeping/Files
☐ Home Models
☐ Labeling
☐ Advance Administration
☐ Fire/Safety/Health
☐ Human Rights/Resident
 Rights
☐ Attitudes
☐ Educational/Vocational
 Programs
☐ Budgeting
☐ Gaming—Handling Situations
 and Behaviors
☐ Medications
☐ Seizures
☐ Academic Development
☐ Normalization
☐ Staff Roles/Job Descriptions
☐ Labor Laws
☐ Use of Volunteers
☐ Insurance
☐ Group Sessions for Residents
☐ Birth Control/Sterilization/
 Abortion
☐ Leisure Time/Recreation
 Programs
☐ Marriage Considerations
☐ Discharge Policies
☐ License Regulations/
 Standards
☐ Assessment Planning
☐ Speech
☐ Physical Therapy
☐ Sign Language
☐ Normal Child Development
☐ Emergency Procedures

☐ Dental Care
☐ Principles of Learning
☐ Changing Behavior
☐ Toilet Training
☐ Special Education
☐ Advocacy
☐ Special Adaptive Equipment
☐ Integration into Community
   Resources
☐ Group Home Evaluations
☐ Food Preparation/Ordering
☐ Other

---

retardation, 2) maintaining healthy environments, 3) fire and safety standards and procedures, 4) administrative responsibilities, 5) elements to be considered in programming, and 6) normalization. These topics seemed to encompass the fundamental understandings we expected from foster parents and group home operators. They also were the topics most frequently mentioned as either being important to the home provider or the client in our survey.

To prepare participants, we send workbooks to everyone in advance of classes. They include the six topic outlines, an introduction to each session, a statement regarding why it is important, specific learning objectives for participants, a list of presenters and their credentials, a comment on what can be expected from them, references, and 10 discussion stimulants for each topic. Participants are also given information on when and where training will be held, when coffee will be served, when the breaks will occur, and so forth. We wanted to get rid of meeting in church basements, institution cafeterias, or inservice rooms. We specifically sought out community colleges as sites because we thought their atmosphere would be beneficial. The community colleges wouldn't help us write the curriculum, but they would let us use their classrooms. This collegiate setting lent a new air of legitimacy and learning to our training sessions. We wanted our training to be powerful, to be respected, to concentrate on subjects recognized as crucial to human services, to have very important documents included, and to be held in a setting readily accepted as a forum for education so that participants would look on the program as being a very serious matter.

Although the entire Macomb-Oakland community placement program is founded on ideology, normalization, and corollary principles, most actual learning objectives for training are practically oriented, not theoretical. For example, in the section on fire and safety considerations, one objective for the participants is, "Describe the most desirable manner to extinguish fires of paper, cloth, wood, grease, gasoline, lighter or cleaning fluids and assorted chemicals." Objectives like these help service providers to respond to a crisis before the crisis occurs. We don't want a fire to start and have people burned because no one knew how to put it out. Here is another example of a practical objective: "What is the first thing you would do upon discovering a fire in progress on a stairway leading to an occupied second floor? What's the second, third, fourth?" Questions like these, it is likely, would never be considered until it was too late.

The discussion stimulants are very important too because they help break up the monotony of didactic sessions with simulation experiences. For example, during the normalization session, we ask people to step in front of the class and role play problem situations. To illustrate: "A hardware store owner wants to give a swing set to a group home for six men. How would you deal with this? Would you call him a fool or would you educate him?"

Written references are probably the least valued element to the participants. Although we list the primary literature sources that our session contents are drawn from on the outline for each session, participants are not typically apt to go out and retrieve the readings from some library. So we bring in copies of the things we think are the most important and distribute them as reprints. Frankly, I am not sure if they're ever read, but even if they are not, I think the references help add more legitimacy to our training program.

## Mandatory Training

We also decided in those early planning days that training would not be voluntary nor time limited. It had to be mandatory and ongoing. It wasn't going to be 6 weeks and it's over, or 100% on three exams and it's over. Training had to be compulsory and forevermore. In the Macomb-Oakland training program, whether a foster parent works for 5 or 10 years does not diminish his or her training attendance responsibility. It is mandatory that he or she come to training sessions on a monthly basis. We write contracts with providers for the payment of services to clients who require room, board, supervision, and in-house programming. The contract also demands monthly attendance at training sessions. If you don't want to come to the training program, we cannot do business. It's not much more complex than that. We were told by many professionals that if we wrote this kind of an expectation into our contracts people would not be interested in providing community placements. But we took the chance, and it has paid off handsomely. We want our service providers to be knowledgeable. We want them to know more about first aid and more about behavior management than most social workers, more than our consultants. We want them to be experts. There is nothing to gain from our wanting anything less. We don't want people who are not interested in taking part in training. We don't feel that we need them. We don't want professionals who are threatened by individuals on their caseload knowing more than they do. We don't feel that we need them.

## Training Costs

It is important to know the costs of our training program because people so often say that what prevents their putting on a good program is that they don't have Title XX money for training or they don't have a grant for the purpose or they cannot pay speakers through normal or abnormal budgetary means. Our training program does not cost anything. Nobody gets paid. There is no special financing, yet the program is excellent.

In the past, we have heard it said countless times that since there's no money, we just can't do it. How are you going to ask a fire marshall, for example, to come in and teach your staff fire prevention for free time after time after time? The answer is simple: you don't ask the same fire marshall each time! We ask favors and we do favors in return. We beg and borrow professional courtesies and it hasn't strained our relationships with colleagues because they view the program with respect and know how much we value their contribution to it. You tell me how many times a fire marshall would otherwise see his name in a printed introduction of a lecture series as someone who attended the Oklahoma Fire College and completed 8 weeks of asbestos training in Ypsilanti, Michigan. Tell me when that man is ever going to be held in as much respect as he is by those 20 service providers who want to know how to put out grease fires. The man is going to come to your session with pride and enthusiasm, not mere resignation, and he is going to turn your participants on to learning important things— if you treat him right.

We've never paid a cent to anybody to conduct a training session. The closest we ever come to paying is buying hungry and thirsty speakers a hamburger and a beer after a training class. If speakers say they can't come back, we ask "Who can replace you? Can you tell us who can come in?" If they say, "I don't know," we say, "Look, we're in this together, you are part of it whether you participate or not." "Do you want it to end?" "We're counting on you to help us." That's not very professional, is it? It's not very dignified either, I realize that. It puts you in a rather compromising position. Who wants to ask for favors? On the other hand, the alternative is even less attractive.

## Training Incentives

There are many incentives for the participants at our training sessions. The self-respect for having acquired knowledge that they get from training is an important consideration. They also receive something else that's subtle, but important: recognition. We have been very fortunate in our agency to receive a lot of positive publicity. We have had people come from hundreds of places across the country, and a few from other parts of the world because they have heard of the Macomb-Oakland Regional Center. When visitors arrive, like Allan Roeher from Canada, we take them out to see our foster parents. We tell our foster parents who he is and how important he is. Knowing that we are so proud of our community placements that we are pleased to show them off to visitors makes people feel pretty good about themselves and the work they are doing. How much does it cost? Nothing! It doesn't cost a cent, but this recognition is a very powerful incentive.

We have a disincentive as well. If you don't come to a training meeting, you lose the money you would ordinarily receive for providing in-house programming for a resident on that day, which usually amounts to about $10. This has only happened a few times without a legitimate reason. Although the situation has never occurred, if a foster parent missed three consecutive training sessions, he or she would be discontinued in the program. We would remove all clients from their service setting.

## TRAINING STRENGTHS AND WEAKNESSES

Our training program has many strengths and some weaknesses. Its weaknesses include the potential to lose creativity and daily initiative. It is, for example, easy to become unimaginative in putting together learning objectives and in selecting resource people to make presentations. It is very easy to become lazy, and we have to constantly check ourselves against it.

It is also easy to excuse absences. "She had to go shopping, could not get a sitter," etc. At Macomb-Oakland, we believe that you have to be very ambitious; you have to sell the value of training to the people who attend. This is a critical factor. The participants have to appreciate the relevance of training content. We want them to know what to do when someone breaks a bone. They must know! It is very easy for social workers and others who put on training programs to take content, approach, and the effect of their own attitude for granted.

Our provider readiness training has allowed us to be aggressive in developing alternative programs. We prepare people to take the toughest kinds of clients; we teach them how to deal with these folks and we pay them fairly for their efforts. We make them accountable for their services, and we are accountable for ours.

Training also helps natural parents become infinitely more secure about community placement, and this is extremely important. It has been our experience that natural parents often view institutions as at least acceptable because they offer a kind of security in their citadel-like appearance, in their predictability. These parents also find comfort in the knowledge that institutional attendants "know" what they are doing. They have been trained. They might be understaffed and so forth, but they have acquired the special skills necessary to work with "mentally retarded" persons.

Because of our extensive training programs, we can now offer natural parents the same kind of security. Now we can say that our foster parents and group home personnel come to the job with more than good intentions and energy. They know what is expected of them and they are prepared to satisfy our expectations. Our foster parents and group home staff know what they are doing, believe me. This knowledge makes service providers and parents, as well as bureaucrats, more confident in the placement program.

Another subject that is important to placement success is language. Our professional jargon can be of benefit when we are discussing concepts with one another, but it can inhibit communication with people who have an interest in our field but are not part of it. People hear the jargon but are not privy to the translation.

We take pains to make sure that jargon used in human services—the acronyms, the abbreviations, the technical terms—are not foreign to our community service providers. When we ask a foster parent to work on a behavior management program, we want them to be familiar with the methods, the technological means as well as the long range goals. We make an effort to be certain that that foster parent knows what we are talking about. It becomes incumbent upon us to interest the provider in the monthly training sessions, to teach them what is involved in working toward behavior management objectives.

A fundamental understanding of the Macomb-Oakland Regional Center training effort is that we, agency professionals, are responsible for the education of foster parents and group home personnel. This tenet places the burden for client habilitation squarely on an identified agency and equally identifiable individuals within it.

Good training of providers virtually eliminates the phenomenon of clients returning to the institution because he or she failed to adjust.

The acceptance of the importance of training and the placement agency's responsibility to provide it places the burden on the right people. Training makes social workers and case managers stay sharp, makes in-house programming possible, allows us to pay foster parents and group home employees adequately, permits us to serve larger numbers of clients, interests more potential providers, makes parents more confident, and accelerates the client's movement toward independence. As we improve our training efforts, our efforts to prepare people who are part of the community placement scene, we increase the quality and the quantity of residential options to the institution. Ambitious provider training and successful community placements are inseparable.

## CONCLUDING COMMENTS

There are additional considerations that have been important to the community placement success we have achieved at Macomb-Oakland. First, when we set out with the notion of making institutional life obsolete, we did not begin by trying to alter the manner in which "mentally retarded" persons were being treated in the entire world, the United States, or even Michigan; just two counties. We began with something, an area and population, that we thought was manageable. Second, we decided that we were going to try to change, not merely improve, the system as it existed. In this regard, we felt that we could patch up the system in a number of places, make a few modifications here and there, and provide a service that most consumers would find acceptable, but not a service that we as professionals with high expectations of ourselves and our resource capability could find acceptable. An improved system that is wrong in its focus is in need of change, not improvement. We committed ourselves to changing the focus. We felt that virtually all "mentally retarded" persons could live nicely in the larger community, so we established a goal of proving that the traditional institution was unnecessary. In keeping with this goal, we decided to work toward two key objectives: 1) returning 100 people per year from institutions to individually preferable residences within their home communities, and 2) having no new institutional admissions. A third very important early consideration was our decision to attack the attitude, or the assumption, that people living in institutions have to "learn" their way out. In 1972, when we went to an out-of-state institution and asked who was ready for community placement, the number didn't require a dozen moves. Hardly anybody was ready! They weren't ready because they hadn't been toilet trained, or they didn't know how to eat independently, or they couldn't dress themselves, or they had maladaptive behavior. They hadn't learned enough to leave.

If you will look, as we did a couple of years ago, at the professional literature and compare the attention shown to preparing retarded people to move out of institutions versus those dealing with the preparation of people who receive the institution's graduates, the ratio is alarming. Over the last 5 years, myriad articles have dealt with preparing clients to become competent enough to leave institutions. Three have treated the subject of provider readiness. There has been an unforgivable lack of attention focused on teaching foster parents, natural parents, group home people, volunteers, administrators, managers, and similarly employed people how to provide human management services in community settings.

We simply decided that we were not going to impose traditional readiness criteria on our institution's residents any more.

We no longer required clients to learn their way out. We thus eliminated an enormous quasi-legitimate barrier. We dumped it! We decided to place training emphasis at the other end of things.

A final factor that seems crucial from our experience was to establish a core group of workers strongly committed to two values: 1) a sense of urgency, and 2) a sense of responsibility.

We have never had more than seven full-time staff members developing placements and organizing training. We continue to meet frequently to reinforce one another's sense of urgency toward our mission. We remind each other that what we are working on has to be done yesterday, that we are writing history, and that we are making major contributions to future trends.

Numbers are important. If there are 1,400 people living, for all practical purposes, like non-citizens in one of our state institutions, they all deserve to come out. Not just seven in a perfect group home that meets all the normalization specifications. They *all* have to come out. We decided that we would do everything possible to create ideal living arrangements for every client, but our inability to create the ideal would not unnecessarily delay the return to the community of any individual living inappropriately within the institution. This sense of urgency is essential; people must be continuously reminded that the people depending upon the products of our labor will not live another lifetime.

By a sense of responsibility, I mean simply that you have to personally accept the obligation to make changes in the system. You and I have this responsibility. We do well to begin by identifying the impediments to change. Are they procedures and policies? If so, we must change the procedures and policies. These changes are made by you personally getting on committees, you personally writing letters, you personally bugging your boss, you personally having him bug his boss, you personally going to interagency meetings, setting up your own training program, putting the arm on people, or going a more diplomatic route, but convincing people to make positive contributions to your program.

We decided that we would never succeed as individuals or as an agency by saying things can't be changed because "that is how the system is." In what is perhaps a melodramatic fashion, we characterize ourselves as revolutionaries who have taken an oath to bring about critical changes in our interagency system and our fellow citizen's system of values.

It is a beautiful, thrilling thing to take on an almost impossible task of changing entrenched practices. The fanaticism flows. The job is so awesome, so outrageous, and yet at the same time so challenging, so invigorating, so poetic, so romantic. You might look at this and other ways we have accomplished things at Macomb-Oakland and judge some of our methods as unconventional or undignified. The fact of the matter is, however, that we have decided that traditional, professional behavior is just not suited to contemporary problems. We have decided to simply use methods that will work for our clients. In doing this, we have sometimes traded the conventional dignity of the professional for the ultimate dignity of the "mentally retarded" citizen. This has seldom proved a bad bargain.

## QUESTIONS AND ANSWERS

QUESTION: Does the increased staff ratio in your foster homes over the institution make a significant difference in an individual's progress?

PROVENCAL: It makes a dramatic difference in the progress of the person who is now living in the community. The person who moves from the institution to the community gets 2 hours a day of training in the home. In addition, he or she attends school, a workshop, or a job in the community. An institution is not conducive to this kind of mobility. Additionally, in a foster home, you don't have a 1:4 or 1:8 ratio, you have one family to a maximum of three clients. Our average is 1.2 people living in each community training home, so it's relatively easy to devote 2 hours a day to tutoring.

QUESTION: Do you deliver the non-core classes in the same way as the core classes, and would you teach something like yoga?

PROVENCAL: Yes, we deliver the non-core classes the same way. If we had enough interest among people attending the inservice, we would bring in a yoga person, but it would just be a one-shot deal.

QUESTIONS: Did you say that your foster home cost is $25 per diem and that you could have three people at $60 a day?

PROVENCAL: Our total cost is approximately $25 per day per client. This includes administrative costs as well. Foster parents receive approximately $20.00 per day per resident. Three residents would earn $60.00 for a foster parent. We think that we place enough demands on the foster parents that the money is well earned. The cost of institutional placements in Michigan averages from $55 a day. Macomb-Oakland supported institutional slots cost over $100.00 per day. It is a bargain any way you look at it, and the quality of placement is just not comparable to the institutional placement.

QUESTION:   Our rates are much lower than that. How can we do it?

PROVENCAL:   Our programs were built on $11 a day per client for the total program. The new rates were a reward to us last year because we were doing such a good job. You can do it by deciding that you have to.

QUESTION:   What about recidivism?

PROVENCAL:   I mentioned that we've had 18 admissions, and that includes readmissions. However, we do have options. For example, take the person who acts out, say a large man who behaves in an aggressive fashion. We can send staff members into his group home, maybe using the same staff from back in the institution. This person might talk to the client, walk him around the block, or write out a new behavioral plan. We would have to do it when he came back, so why not try it before then? The other thing we can do is explore another placement for him. If he's got to move, let's look at some other community homes. Some people might say that moving him from one home to another is unsettling. It's a lot less unsettling to move a person from one group home to another than from a group home to an institution. These approaches have been very effective for keeping people out of institutions. Almost totally! I mentioned we have had 18 admissions. These mostly came in the first 2 or 3 years when we had few supports to rely on.

QUESTION:   Do you use group homes and your community training facilities for your medically fragile, multiply handicapped as well?

PROVENCAL:   Yes, we do. But we feel a need to expand and improve this service. From time to time when visitors come, they particularly want to see if we're talking about really highly dependent, multiply handicapped people moving into the larger community. We haven't placed as many people who are medically fragile as we would like, but we have placed many such people. This group makes up the largest part of the people who are remaining in institutions.

QUESTION: What about babies?

PROVENCAL: We're very fortunate in Michigan. Since 1972, we've had an extremely progressive special education law, which really took off about 3 years ago. We have mandatory special education for everybody from ages 0 to 26. Now, not all districts are performing, but since it is on the books, parents are educating themselves about the services due their child. The result has been that we have very few requests for infant services.

QUESTION: Do you have the same kind of programs for the people in the pediatric nursing homes that you have for the others?

PROVENCAL: It isn't the identical program. It is closer to an institutional program because it's more medically oriented. Nurses run it almost exclusively. We haven't given this sufficient attention as yet.

QUESTION: What sort of cooperation do you get from the parents of people you are placing out of institutions?

PROVENCAL: It really has gone up dramatically. In the last 5 years, we've only had one parent resist us right down the line on community placement. We've had hundreds disapprove in the beginning, but we get other parents to support us. We've made the parents who are most in favor of our program into salespeople. When parents resist, we ask our supportive parents to speak with those who are resisting. They are our best ambassadors. Who wants to listen to a social worker like me tell a parent what he or she should do with a son or daughter? What do I know about matters of their heart, their guilt, their desire for protection? How could I know? Other parents know and they can be extremely helpful during the deliberation.

QUESTION: What would you do if the state decided to expand the types of handicapped people you serve?

PROVENCAL: I don't think it would make much difference to us whether they expand, as appears to be the case, the definition of those eligible for service. It will give us a new group to serve and we will have to learn some new things. The critical point is that we are committed to providing alternatives to institutions. If group homes and workshops are too institutional, the next movement must be to change them. I think we can replicate with other disability categories the things that we have learned through working predominantly with "mentally retarded" persons. We have been approached by groups like United Cerebral Palsy and the Epilepsy Foundation to help develop segregated group homes.

We've declined to participate. Segregated, exclusive homes for these populations would be easy to do, but wrong. Instead, we have provided these groups help in developing more integrated services.

We've developed 30 group homes in 4½ years. Now we know that we have too many group homes. We still don't have enough people out of institutions, but we have developed too many group homes. We don't want to create more segregated services, even group homes. We have to go further. If your group approached us with a desire to develop residential alternatives for autistic children, we'd probably help you set up foster homes, with the foster parents trained in accordance with our community training home model, or help you work with natural parents in some similar capacity.

QUESTION: What kinds of experiences, if any, have you had with community resistance?

PROVENCAL: We've had quite a variety of experience concerning community resistance. I have several opinions about it.  One is that it's very easy to get turned off and have your efforts blunted because you've raised the ire of property owners. We've been turned down in asking for zoning exceptions a dozen times. We have had bloody battles and we've had battles where there was no bloodletting whatsoever. Sometimes you cannot even tell who your opponents are. We also have had some wonderful experiences where we've been able to turn around entire neighborhoods. Occasionally, when a provider vendor has found an especially good home, we have been able to go and talk to the neighbors and tell them the difference between our clients and what they think they are. Many people, for example, still confuse "mentally ill" and "mentally retarded" individuals. They take the most extreme examples of one category and apply it to the most general member of the other category.

It is an easy, obvious excuse not to open a home because property owners will not let you into their neighborhood. But there are all kinds of neighborhoods out there where they will accept you. If you happen to pick on a neighborhood where the zoning isn't right, there are other neighborhoods around. There are millions of homes in our area. Why get turned off entirely because one group turns you off? Anyway, it may be a blessing in disguise. As Wade Hitzing says, "We shouldn't have six sailors or six chorus girls living together." Why fault the community? Let's start working toward only having one and two people living together. That's what we should all be about anyway.

We also have an obligation to do a number of other things. One is that we have to continually educate everyone and not just the guy who is trying to fight us. Macomb-Oakland Regional Center makes an all-out attempt to influence newspapers, and we make sure that they print what we want by sending them newsworthy stories that are positively oriented. We frequently make contacts with reporters for the purpose of educating them to our goals, our problems, and our needs. We've made a very concerted effort to do these things, and we have hundreds of positive articles printed every year.

QUESTION: I don't see how we could replicate your program in Los Angeles. It's too big. Our hospitals have thousands of people in them.

PROVENCAL: We are dealing with hundreds of people in our catchment area. Without question, your problem is much larger. Some of us had an opportunity to work in New York on the Willowbrook Plan. They told us that we "white-socked hicks" from the Midwest could in no way understand the "Big Apple," and that our service concepts really should be left in the boondocks. Willowbrook's problems were considered too complex. They kept talking about the bilingual problem, the Staten Island Ferry, and other things that we really didn't have any understanding of. But we decided that the principles we had were universal, and that the program concepts we had, although they weren't terribly novel, had any number of variations. For example, if it's not a group home for eight people, why not have a group home for four, or why not apartments? Why not look to apartment owners? I understand Philadelphia, Pennsylvania has been a pioneer in making use of apartments. Why not have your social workers go around and visit people in their apartments? Why not develop core residential units where you have one group home that supervises people living in their own apartments scattered around the city? There are people who are a lot more imaginative than I am who can devise any number of residential concepts to meet your needs. Macomb-Oakland is moving away from traditional group homes. We are looking for better things. We would still open a group home to get eight persons out of an institution, but we would rather see program models that are more normative.

In any case, there are answers for Los Angeles. You just have to look for them.

# BEYOND THE FAMILY AND THE INSTITUTION
## The Sanctity of Liberty

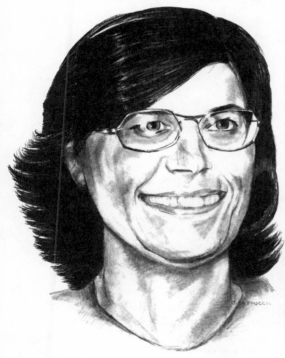

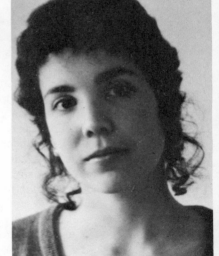

Betty Pieper and
Joanna Cappuccilli

## RESIDENTIAL ISSUES FOR THE FAMILY

*N*ot long ago, there were only two ways in which society sought to manage people with noticeable disabilities: put them in institutions or ignore them within their families. Both solutions often felt like punishment. Those families who chose institutions were actively encouraged not to visit or become attached to their offspring. Alternately, those who kept their children at home struggled quietly out of sight in the community with the crushing care, expense, and social isolation that are still common. In the following pages, we point out the serious issues that must be addressed in order to make the changes needed to improve the plight of the family. We present some strategies for exercising familial rights. We offer a way to use a modern philosophy, an examination of bureaucratic manipulation, and residential alternatives to fight for.

The general public viewed disability as a stigma on a family. The prevailing, if unconscious, attitude was that disabilities represented a fall from grace, an outward sign of an inward blemish, and, in general, one's just desserts. People didn't want to meddle with divine judgment to provide relief. Eugenic theorists were afraid to treat such people too kindly for fear of encouraging those with inferior genes to produce more disabilities and thus contaminate our gene pool. All of these attitudes are alive and well today, although they may be presented in slightly different guises, and all of these attitudes have an ever-present effect on the family with a member who is disabled.

Public exposure of terrible abuses within institutions during the 1960s brought forth legal suits. Courts held that institutionalized people had a right to treatment in the least restrictive setting possible. Concurrently, the Civil Rights Movement made the public, including parents, conscious of issues like due process, segregation, and non-elected political power of privileged groups who could literally buy control of people's lives.

Out of a rash of legal suits we have discovered how emotionally charged and how complex the issue of where and how people live really is. People have become polarized, faction fighting faction. The bureaucracy that previously discouraged home care is now encouraging distant relatives to take in grown family members so that it can meet court-ordered decrees to deinstitutionalize a certain number of people. However, funding sources still give incentive to state institutions and private institutional nursing homes, and other sections of the law give only lip service to community services and less restrictive settings.

Standards tend to be based upon beds and floor space rather than more relevant criteria, and doctors still tend to be in charge of developmental concerns when their training is not in these areas at all. Worst of all, this inappropriate management model threatens to spread into the community despite its abysmal failure behind institutional walls. Powerful lobbies have convinced the government that, because a person has an ongoing medical problem, it should dominate his whole life, and all living activities should revolve around this aspect of the person. This is about the same as saying that since I sleep nearly a third of my life, the AMM (American Mattress Manufacturers) should decide where I live, with whom, and what I eat.

> Experience should teach us to be most on our guard to protect liberty when the government's purposes are beneficient. The greatest dangers to liberty lurk in insidious encroachment by men of zeal, well-meaning but without understanding (Justice Brandeis in *Olmstead* v. *U.S.*) (1)

Until recently, it was believed that people with disabilities were not fully human and therefore not citizens of standing like other people. One has only to read old documents in order to understand that mentally retarded and physically handicapped people were regarded as deviant and tainted. In many cases laws that forbid these people to appear in public are still on the books.

Because of these beliefs, the government could and did act under the "parens patriae" principle derived from old English law, which named the King as guard or guardian. The government could then define the ward's welfare as it saw fit and convenient. Furthermore, the doctrine of state's interest allowed that the populace could be protected from whatever or whomever it considered morbid, disgusting, or even inconvenient. Only recently, as beliefs change, are the rights and needs of disabled people and their families being looked at and measured in relation to those of valued citizens.

## Normalization

In order to be effective agents of change, we must believe in a philosophy that will give us guidelines for implementing an improved service system. Although widely misunderstood, normalization is one principle that does, if properly used, provide a model for changing outdated systems. It is a valuable tool for evaluating every service setting. The principle holds that every service setting must be designed to use culturally typical means to secure a valued image for people with disabilities, at least as good as other citizens of the same age.

Normalization makes use of some of the most significant and empirically demonstrated principles in the field of learning. People learn by seeing others doing tasks. Therefore, a disabled person, although generally devalued, can also learn by observing a generally valued person doing a task, and that task can be broken down into simple steps that will allow a mentally or physically limited person to achieve success. People learn best by actually doing a task and experiencing the accomplishment involved. Also, a person is *more* motivated to do tasks he or she sees as useful than an artificially created curriculum isolated from real life; and a skill is learned better and is retained longer when it is used as part of real life routinely.

Another important principle of learning is that the expectations of others tend to be fulfilled, so that if we expect competence we are more likely to get it. A person's self-image affects his or her ability to learn, so it is important to be conscious of what we say. We need to avoid calling people names like *retardate, cripple, patient,* or *MR.* We must also remember that the variety and scope of experience affect learning. Experiences are usually richer and broader in integrated settings.

Normalization seeks to have a person develop to his or her best potential. The support system needed for this development consists of specialized components developed in the context of the same community agencies that serve all people. Separate and segregated programs should not exist. For example, an interpreter of sign language should sign a public address at an open meeting instead of delivering a speech at another time for deaf people. A mentally disabled person should be welcomed for medical treatment in the same facilities as other citizens.

Normalization requires that rhythms of life be respected. All activities should not be viewed as treatment and occur within a given building. In the morning an adult goes to work and a child to school. Recreation ought to take place in modified programs of local parks and community centers. Most children live with their families. Most adults want to live independently or at least choose their own place of residence. People develop companionship ties and many marry and raise children. Parents, after raising their children, look forward to the time when they can be free to travel, move to smaller quarters, or otherwise have time to themselves. They maintain a relationship with their offspring in a new manner.

## Normalization and Civil Rights for Parents

There is a point of unity that may yet bind relatives and friends of the disabled into a powerful political force. It is that we want the best for our disabled family member as well as *protection for ourselves.* Our fear of being responsible for more care, expense, responsibility, and emotional stress than we can bear prevails upon us. Likewise we realize, at some unconscious level, that we and our children will never be truly valued members of society until all punitive responses toward us are eradicated. We aspire to be publicly vindicated of a crime we never committed. We want to be treated as other citizens are. We want to be protected from undue restriction of our personal freedom and from excessive demands on our financial resources.

Somehow, few parents have admitted such feelings publicly. Good parents are expected to carry their cross without complaining even when their backs are broken from the weight; and these parents, true to societal pressures, go on without speaking out for themselves for fear people will continue to question their children's worth. One mother wrote to *The Exceptional Parent* (2):

> I have just finished reading "The Dark Side" and feel slight relief that there are some parents who also hate. After 12 guilt-ridden years of searching for medical help, an education and a place in society, I feel we can no longer help her. She did not respond. We do not love her nor does she love us. I will take care of her but I cannot fulfill the requirement of loving her.

In the December, 1977 issue of this same magazine, a woman tells of being asked to care for a brother who had been institutionalized all of his life. She remarked, "I don't know whether I need a psychologist or a lawyer" (3). As might be expected, she was afforded psychological treatment to "help work through her feelings about her brother." The state and federal policies that are currently wreaking havoc with people's lives went unquestioned. Unless we are willing to see the issues clearly and challenge policies that violate our rights, no permanent relief or justice can come.

In its extreme haste to depopulate institutions, under court order, our government has forgotten that parents and relatives also have rights. Relatives must not be taken advantage of to accommodate either changing social policy or to facilitate the easy way out for bureaucracies. The care of a severely disabled child is extremely restrictive of a caregiver's freedom. It is certainly fair to expect people who have children with special needs to take responsibility for them *up to the level they would encounter for a typical child,* but it is punitive to require more. In many families, it is no exaggeration to call the consequences cruel and unusual punishment for all concerned. All of this happens without a formal charge being brought or any due process occurring. Ironically, a woman would have more personal freedom today if she had been accused of a heinous crime 16 years ago rather than if she gave birth today to a child with a severe disability.

It is particularly unfair to expect parents and relatives to be primary caregivers after a disabled family member reaches 18 years of age. Other citizens in this society are not responsible for their adult offspring and equal protection under the law demands that parents of individuals with special needs be treated no differently. However, because of their own feelings of guilt and protection, many parents feel they have this responsibility for life. Reasonable alternatives have been designed for providing services to disabled adults. It is time they were implemented.

Does all of this sound like some parents want to get rid of their children or to have nothing further to do with them? It is not meant to. No family wants that. What they want is freedom to relate to their disabled children as they would to other children. One does not give up loving, worrying, advising, or seeing offspring because they move out of their physical homes. Families get together in times of sickness or sorrow, to celebrate special occasions, or share vacations. Parents may even give help with down payments on homes or buying expensive presents if they can afford to. These are typical relationships.

These types of relationships not only benefit parents, but also their children. Since parents often expect to care for their children even as adults, they often restrict their children from becoming more independent. However, if times were changed, and parents automatically expected typical life-styles for their children, more parents would be willing to let go. Disabled people have voiced it over and over again that overprotective attitudes have limited their development and exposure.

By heeding our own self-interest instead of feelings of martyrdom, parents could join with disabled adults in demanding settings that give both of us freedom and fully protect our rights. It is not typical or particularly valued for adults to live in their parents' homes, unless one chooses this as a long-term arrangement. What we have to do is understand the possible stigma attached, and be certain the choice is made consciously and willingly, out of preference and not for lack of an alternative arrangement.

The threat of being alone without assistance has forced parents into accepting extremes—the family forever, the massive institutions, or the nursing home. Parents have accepted poor services because they believed they had no recourse and no alternative. What if parents forced the issue by banding together for specific goals? What if the federal government said that service settings that violate disabled people's rights are out, and a lack of service is not an option either because it violates family rights? Can't we demand residential settings and a comprehensive system of services?

## Useful Normalization Questions

Wolf Wolfensberger and Linda Glenn, acknowledged leaders in services for people with disabilities, have created an assessment tool for judging the degree of normalization in a service setting. The rating instrument is called *Program Analysis of Service Systems,* or PASS (4). PASS training is very rigorous and requires several weeks of workshops and supervised practice before a rater is qualified. Without this specialized training, however, one can easily begin to recognize appropriate versus nonappropriate residences. The following are helpful questions, based upon PASS, that can assist one in determining how typical or like most people's dwellings a given residence is. Answering yes to all or many questions means the home is likely to be an appropriate setting.

1. Did the residents choose to live in the home? It is important, to the extent possible, that people live where they *choose* to live and not necessarily where they were placed.
2. Is this the type of setting usually inhabited by people in the resident's age group? For example, it is not appropriate for a young child to live in a convalescent home.
3. Do the residents live with others their own age? It is not appropriate, other than within a family context, for children and adults to live together. A great deal of one's socialization skills and interpersonal interaction is from peers, and roommates generally choose age mates for companionship.
4. Is the residence located within a residential neighborhood? It is important for adequate integration and improved public attitude that people who are already valued in society live nearby. It is better not to have the residence isolated in the country or, worse yet, in a business or industrial district.
5. Does the residence look like the other dwellings around it? It is important that the building fit the neighborhood. It should not look like a monument, hospital, or shack. It should look like the typical housing within the area. It should also not have a name on it. It only needs a simple street address like other people's homes. Institutional symbols, such as firebells and exit signs, should not be used. They only tell people the home is different.
6. Can the number of people living in the residence be reasonably expected to assimilate into the community? In other words, if children and foster parents live in the home, their

number must be the same as one would expect from a typical family. If adults live in a group, there must not be more than a typical group of roommates in one dwelling. Large crowds draw attention. It is important to keep the size manageable so that the neighbors aren't overwhelmed with a situation they can't learn to accept. It is also important that the residents have enough valued people around them to emulate and to help them feel like accepted citizens.

7. Are community resources and facilities readily accessible from the residence? It is crucial that the person be able to get to community facilities. They must be close enough, and there must be adequate transportation readily available.

8. Do the residents have a chance to buy the house? The people who live in a house or apartment that can be bought should have a chance to buy it if they have the funds. Their money should not be spent in their name for the employment of staff members or for purchase by an agency. Sometimes inheritances are given people, or parental investments for their children are made. These investments could be put into the home in the resident's name so that it becomes his or her own home and shuffling around because of any agency changes would end. Or, if the person chose to move elsewhere, his or her share of the investment should move, too.

9. Do the managers of the place act in an appropriate manner toward the residents? There are many factors to consider here. The most important is that the staff members treat people under their supervision with dignity and respect. If the residents are adults, staff members should not call them boys or girls, or in any other way display undue power. An assistant or associate role is preferable to a parental role. Staff members should also not act as if they own the place. If the managers also live in the residence, they should consider it a living arrangement and not merely a place to work. They should feel comfortable inviting their personal friends over because they consider it their home, too.

10. Are the residents encouraged to do all they can for themselves? Residents must have full access to laundry machines, all kitchen equipment, and other household and garden appliances. As much as possible each person must be encouraged to prepare food and care for their clothing and house. The most powerful learning is doing, and being able to increase one's independence.

11. Are the residents encouraged to have personal belongings that are appropriate to their ages? Adults should not have toys, furniture, or other materials that label them childlike or excessively dependent. Belongings should enhance one's individuality. Barren rooms or uniform clothes and accessories are inappropriate and stigmatizing.

12. Are residents encouraged to use community resources as much as possible? The residence should not be sufficient unto itself. To the extent that they are able, residents should learn to bank, shop, and use community businesses. They should have access to generic medical services without living in a "medicalized" setting. They should be encouraged to learn to use emergency services, such as the fire department and police. They should learn to use the telephone and public transportation. They should work and go to school in the community with everyone else.

13. Are all the residents' rights acknowledged? Residents must have privacy when they wish. They must have freedom from unnecessary medical attention. They must be allowed to receive mail, use the phone, and have visitors. Adults should be allowed to set their own hours. There are community services available to assist people in identifying and maintaining these and other rights.

14. Are the residents being given enough training and assistance to help them be competent, growing, developing individuals? A disability should not prevent anyone from being given enough assistance to grow and change. Some accommodations should be made to promote development in each resident to the extent that he or she is able.

15. Would I want to live in the home? Here is the final test. If the residence appears good enough for you to want to live in it, it will probably be an appropriate living arrangement for persons with special needs. We should demand residential arrangements for persons with special needs that are comparable to those inhabited by most nondisabled citizens.

## MONUMENTAL MYTHS

Normalization is often misinterpreted and misused. People frequently fail to realize that it is merely a tool for improving man's humanity toward man. Properly understood it gives us guidelines upon which to build improved services for our fellow citizens. There are six prevailing myths regarding normalization.

## "Normalization Means Neglect of Intellectual and Social Development"

Professional journals are full of critics of normalization who all say essentially the same thing. Since the community failed the disabled population, it obviously cannot work for them. And if people don't fit into the present structure, they need specialized services rendered in institutional settings. These critics are correct in saying that it will not do to put people back into the same environments that failed them. No true proponent of normalization has ever suggested doing so.

"Dumping" people into communities from institutions without support is not normalization! The normalization principle is greatly concerned with highly specialized support services and clinical/technical expertise, which can be used to help people achieve greater degrees of independence. People who misrepresent normalization in this way are often benefiting from the present system and do not wish change. Two of the most important ratings on PASS are concerned with appropriate clinical or technical skills provided to people and the intensity of appropriate programming in order to increase their skills.

In an institutional setting where programming is medically oriented, all the support services are administered under one roof. The medical model means that children passively receive education, therapy, vocational rehabilitation, and sick care all under the auspices of treatment. It is not uncommon to find that a licensed professional does range of motion exercises for a quarter of an hour and then the child is returned to a crib for the rest of the day.

The disadvantages to this form of living are many. An occupational therapist shows a film on how to wash hands before eating, but the building has no sink low enough for those in wheelchairs to use. A young woman with spina bifida may be counseled by a full-time licensed physician to drink plenty of fluids, but be unable to find a sink, fountain, or refrigerator that is accessible to her or a bathroom that she can use independently. Activities of daily living classes may teach about the four food groups or even how to spread a sandwich, but if there is no opportunity to shop, plan menus, or prepare one's own food, these skills are useless. Speech therapy may be delivered for short periods each day by a licensed therapist, but the person is returned to a ward of people who do not talk and the results are understandably poor. The public may feel comfortable knowing that people with disabilities are being "taken care" of in institutions, but the effects of this type of living are questionable.

The normalization principle suggests, on the other hand, that we must make use of valued, typical means in order to teach skills. Church groups, Y programs, adult education, park recreational programs, libraries, and special interest groups that meet in each other's homes to play cards or sew are typical ways of learning. People with special needs should be allowed access to these activities. Children with disabilities should go to school programs like all other children. Tutors, therapists, and nurses can still be hired if needed. The difference is that, when served in the community, individuals have somewhere to apply the skills they are learning. If these support systems are provided with enough planning, assistance, and counseling, community programs will work.

## "There Will Always Be Those Who Need Institutions"

There may always be people who need special assistance. They may always—despite the best training or medical treatment—need help dressing, eating, or getting around. There may always be people who need special equipment, such as standing tables, respirators, ramps, and grab bars in bathrooms. It may be that some people will always need special programming and individualized plans in order to cope successfully with everyday society. There may be, despite intensive training, people who remain largely dependent upon others throughout their lives, and they do need places to live just as the rest of us do. But by what leap of logic do these needs mean that such persons require institutions as they currently exist? Certainly there are abundant data that suggest that such places are *not* good for meeting these needs, certainly not when compared to a less restrictive environment.

We do not mean to imply that all children should stay with their families. It may be that there are people who cannot afford to remodel their homes or who move too often to allow this. It may be that some parents do not want to give up career goals in order to devote the tremendous amounts of time that some children require. It may be that some people need residences that are specially adapted to their needs, or that cost effectiveness demands that certain services or facilities be shared. These are not reasons why severely disabled people must live out of the public domain, however. As described in other chapters of this book, alternative home environments with the proper supportive services can be created.

It may be more convenient for service providers to congregate people together. It may even be that parents of disabled people will accept facilities based upon the medical model rather than initiate legal struggles or fight extensive bureaucracies. There are many reasons why people promote and accept institutional settings, but human needs can always be served in other ways. Many of the parents at Willowbrook Developmental Center in New York realized this. Although they accepted institutional placement for their own needs, they actively forced the issue so that their children could have their needs met in more typical and valued settings.

## "Parents Who Institutionalize Their Children Are Unnatural Parents and Morally Inferior People— They Have No One to Blame but Themselves if Their Children Are Abused"

Every time there is an exposé of an institutionalized resident being scalded in a shower where he was left unwittingly or brutalized by another resident while left unattended there is a horrible outcry. It is always short-lived, however, and usually a good bit of it turns to, "What kind of people would put their children in such a place?" One legislative aide remarked after the Willowbrook hearings, "Can you imagine? After all this, the waiting list is still increasing!"

Let us be very clear about one thing. No parent ever "put" his or her child into a state institution. The state did that. It was the response parents chose at one point, based upon prevailing public attitudes and the "expert testimony" of medical authorities and others in power. The parents may have given up being able to bear total responsibility, but the state (you and I and a lot of others) decided upon the specific places into which they would "put" people.

It seems easier to put the blame on individuals since something as massive and nebulous as "the state" tends to overwhelm us. We convince ourselves that what is too big to be understood is also benign. It is easier to blame the victims of misfortune for somehow bringing it upon themselves. The truth is that options for parents have been limited and that funding has given incentive to settings that some of us find abhorrent.

## "People with Extensive Medical Involvement Cannot Live in Typical, Normal Settings"

"Medical" is what we define it to be, or rather what the medical establishment defines it to be. If only licensed nurses can own or use needles and syringes for the injection of insulin, then people with diabetes might have to live in nursing homes rather than run out to the doctor's office every day. If catheters can only be possessed by physicians and if instructions or supplies are not available, obviously it is not possible to run out four times a day to a clinic. If the situation is redefined, a person can take care of this intimate need at home. Even an ordinary diaper can become "medical treatment" for incontinence if your doctor prescribes it. Plain things can become "medical" and exotic things can become commonplace if we are open to redefining who can do what and where.

If, on the other hand, doctors make no provision for occasional house calls or continue to practice in inaccessible offices, then at some point the difficulty becomes such that we are forced to use nursing homes for a modicum of care at crucial times. It seems that these facilities are overutilized in order to qualify for care or the payment for care that is otherwise not available.

Today, there are a few good models in the United States where people with severe medical and developmental difficulties live well. Despite their life-threatening conditions, with the proper supportive staffing these people are living comfortably in small settings. Specialists are needed to provide monitoring services. The residents are receiving more individualized care than they would in a large facility, for substantially less cost. Nebraska, Michigan, Minnesota, and Pennsylvania have allocated their resources to develop such programs, and some scattered local efforts exist in other states as well. One such home, recently acclaimed exemplary by a member of the President's Committee on Mental Retardation, is described in a subsequent chapter.

## "There Are Day Programs Available in the Community and Therefore There Are Community Services"

This myth discounts the need for community residential services. Sometimes, for a variety of reasons, it is not appropriate for a child to stay at home with his or her parents. First of all, being in the community does not necessarily mean normal. Nor is it even *necessarily* less dehumanizing or isolating than an institutional setting. We have all heard horror stories of the treatment of children within their own homes that could compare with any institutional abuse. Some parents do not understand the ramifications of their children's disabilities. If the parents are not receptive to learning, alternative living arrangements must be made. By community service, people often mean day programs, and day programs only. However, residential choices are an important dimension of community living. Community living necessitates group homes, adapted apartments within all public housing, itinerant and live-in attendants, accessible private housing in many kinds of neighborhoods, specially adapted travel trailers for vacations, adapted units at resorts used by the general public, specially trained family care parents with accessible homes for respite stays, adapted camping equipment and sites so that youngsters can go on Y trips or Scout outings *with* typical youngsters, and so on. Sufficient places and the creative, flexible arrangements to fill special needs are required in order for disabled people to ever be truly accepted and integrated.

## "More Data Need to Be Collected and More Research Must Be Done to Prove that Normalization and Community Living Can Work"

Critics say that normalization is just a slogan and that empirical evidence is needed before we can change social policy. Yet daily we can see that the old model has consumed our resources in the absence of any evidence that it is humane or cost effective. The question no longer is whether or not to change. That has been decided for us. Social policy is built upon values and beliefs. In the past, people believed that having a disability was evidence of sin, divine judgment, or a fall from grace. They often believed that mental retardation was contagious. Fear and moralistic attitudes brought forth segregation. Now we must set forth new social policy on beliefs and values that hold that differences *should* be accepted, that caring for one another can deepen and enrich us, that people are entitled to be valued for themselves, and that our constitution protects all citizens equally.

All social research is subject to the biases of those conducting it. For example, not long ago a state employees' union published a monograph entitled *Deinstitutionalization: Out of Their Beds and into the Streets* (5). Although the abuses described in this publication were no doubt true, the problems described were the results of unsupported "dumping." The purpose of the monograph was to scare people and save institutional jobs. Normalization advocates can document astounding examples of human growth and personal happiness when people are placed in the community with supports. Although some research may be useful in telling us just what kind of services or settings people need or want, such research is usually done from the perspective of service providers or managers and staff, seldom from the point of view of consumers. We need to be honest in admitting that normalization is based upon values and beliefs about people. It also has vigorous concern with constitutional issues and political rights. It may be supported by research, but it is not dependent upon research for its validity.

### "What Is Normal Anyway, and Isn't It Just as Oppressive to Demand that Disabled People Fit a Certain Mold?"

Normalization does not propose a universal definition of normal. It only says that, within a given culture, there exist generally accepted behavior patterns to which most people adhere. One is not easily accepted within that culture if one does not follow those behaviors. It is our commitment to give disabled people the opportunity and assistance to acquire those behaviors that make him or her accepted. It is also our intention, once this happens, that nondisabled people will become more accepting of disabled people's evident differences.

To force society to give all its citizens equal opportunities, including civil rights and the option to make certain choices, may be considered by some to be oppressive; however, others will recognize it for what it is—a movement for freedom. It is not that this philosophy expects all to fit a certain mold; only that disabled people become enough like other people to be accepted by the whole of society. We cannot expect people to feel the joy of life if they are isolated and rejected.

If disabled people can be given the opportunity to learn culturally accepted behaviors, then we will recognize that everyone can be competent in some way. If you see someone with a severe mental disability performing competently one job on an assembly line, you will be less likely to consider the disability and more likely to value that person as an individual. For too long, the disability has been considered the person. This is extremely dehumanizing and detrimental to a person's development. With growth and accomplishment, the disability is diminished, not erased. It is simply of less value in identifying the person.

## THE UNYIELDING, UNRESPONSIVE SYSTEM

A few years ago a New York Spina Bifida Association received an SOS from parents who had a baby girl with a disability. Apparently, their neighbors had registered a number of complaints regarding inappropriate care of the child. Without an investigation, the child was removed from her home and placed in a foster home with restrictions on parent visitation.

These parents were obviously not treated fairly. A letter was written telling the authorities that, indeed, the care of a child with spina bifida was complex and that many parents would need supportive help. Such help might include training by a visiting nurse, respite care, financial aid, counseling, or babysitting so that the family could take advantage of opportunities to bind itself to the community. These services should have been offered in order to support, rather than supplant, the family.

The letter expressed, as politely as possible, that the family's rights had been violated without due process. Persons can, of course, be deprived of liberty and of property, including their own children, or have their premises searched, but the Constitution outlines safeguards to protect ordinary citizens. The much-quoted Fifth and Fourteenth Amendments say that "no person . . . shall be deprived of life, liberty, or property without due process of law."

For many years due process meant fundamental fairness. Now it has come to require, in addition, specific procedures. Among these are the right to be informed of the charges against you, the right to confront and cross-examine your accusers, the right to an attorney, the right to call witnesses on your own behalf, the right to an impartial trial, and so forth. Unfortunately, some of these safeguards apply to criminals caught in the act of violating person and property, but not to civil cases. It is no wonder that many parents feel that they are treated worse than confessed criminals.

The president of the local spina bifida group called several attorneys and government officials around the state. They were unanimous in saying that a writ of habeas corpus could return the child to her home within 24 hours. Furthermore, they were quite open in saying that a court-appointed attorney would not provide a fair defense because his employment would create conflict of interest. However, no Legal Aid or other attorney was interested and so the family lost their child to foster care 90 miles from their home. It is terribly disheartening to see a child put in a home where money is provided to foster parents for her care without offering the same service to the natural parents.

Incidents such as the one reported are not uncommon. *Amicus,* the official publication of the National Center on Law and the Handicapped, devoted a major portion of its December, 1976 issue to related reports. The magazine quotes Herman Fogata, then Director of the East Los Angeles Regional Center for the Developmentally Disabled, as saying, "Guardianship of a person can be effected without the person whose rights are being taken away having any kind of legal consultation" (6). The same issue tells of a mother who suffered an emotional breakdown from 2 years of a battle for custody of her child whom a social worker suddenly decided needed 24-hour institutional care. *Amicus* reported simply, "The stories are endless."

A Schenectady parent expressed the anger that parents can feel who are not threatened with the loss of their children, but who are nonetheless violated by laws that give support to out-of-home settings but not to them:

> Our burden is doubly compounded when we read in the newspaper that foster parents receive monthly sums of money, plus year-end allowances to care for these same or less damaged children. Where in our laws has the mistake been made that discriminates against natural parents who want to take care of their own children? How much longer are we going to wait before this injustice gets corrected?" (7)

A mother from New Jersey told *Playboy* (8) her story. Although this may seem an unusual place to find such an outpouring of frustration, it perhaps fell on more sympathetic ears than she had already tried. She wrote, in part:

> Although we would desperately like to care for him at home and give him the love and attention that he couldn't possibly receive in an institution, we can't afford to do so. My husband is a disabled veteran, unable to work, and the small income I bring home is barely enough to meet our basic needs, certainly not enough for the special care Dominick has to have.

The State Bureau of Children's Services has only one solution: to put Dominick into a state institution. We have refused to do so because we feel he would die in an institution and that we could care for him at home. What is crazy about all this is that state officials admit that Dominick's institutionalization would cost the taxpayers more than $8,000 a year. For half that amount, we, his parents, could care for him and save the taxpayers $4,000. [The $8,000 a year figure is a gross misestimate. Today the average annual cost per resident in a state institution is between $18,000 and $40,000.]

Even with systematic violation of human rights and irrational use of public money, most of us cannot afford the kind of action that could change the status of community services. Certainly simply exposing abuse of civil rights and economic resources has not been enough to effect large-scale change. In order to bring about change it is not so necessary to understand the inconsistencies as it is to comprehend who profits from the present model. It is necessary to confront those people and professions who profit at our expense in order to alter the present funding channels. Big business and the medical profession all but control the economic policies of our public institutions, squeezing out the parent or concerning human service worker from consideration.

In many states the profits and patronage in construction and the sale of public bonds dictate expansion of facilities and public policy. The big businesses buy the tax-exempt bond issues and fix public mortgage payment until the cumulative debt service reaches far into the future. Deinstitutionalization is mere rhetoric to the bond holders whose investments must be guarded.

Licensing standards that qualify Title XIX funds from the federal government for matched state dollars command that nurses and doctors be in charge of drugs and treatment. The current movement to reclassify state institutions as "intermediate care facilities" is backed by various special interest groups in an attempt to hold on to the federal Medicaid dollars. If you want your government money, you will have to take our medicine, in other words. Any attempt to switch to a more flexible and integrated model means risking the loss of political monies for decency and justice's sake—hardly a practical course for most bureaucracies. Parents, workers, and clients alike become specks on the implacable and unyielding wall of fiscal and professional dominance and power interests.

The irony is that most of us don't see the real truth. How does a humble citizen or parent discover the truth, and then try to fight city hall? Protest or attack on these hallowed structures antagonizes the employees who, although devoted to the best job they can do, are the thin and sensitive protective skin that defends the unseen skeleton of the system. Key workers, whose jobs depend upon public acceptance of large segregated facilities, howl when parents or enlightened citizens protest.

The fight goes on anyway and sometimes with unsanctioned weapons. As a result of lack of funding resources, a number of quasi-legal schemes have been developed in order to get tax money for natural parents who don't wish out-of-home placement for their children. Two doctors, one with New York State's Department of Mental Hygiene and the other with a clinic for birth defects in Seattle, Washington, have spoken of counseling parents to give up custody of their children. They then re-apply for aid as foster parents or family care for their own children! One professional went so far as to say that parents should divorce so that mothers could receive enough public money to keep their children home.

When people must resort to these actions in order to keep their children out of institutions, something is terribly wrong. Although traditionally a conservative magazine, a *Reader's Digest* article commented upon the "commercial jails" that so many children have been forced into by lack of community support (9):

> The Dyer facility is but one part of a billion dollar industry providing board, shelter, and treatment for some 700,000 children removed from their homes on neglect charges, or yielded up voluntarily by parents who can't cope with their mental retardation or emotional problems.

Add to this the numbers of physically disabled children and adults who are in institutions or nursing homes because there is no more suitable place, and the expense of the industry climbs.

A 1977 HEW report (10) discloses that $272 million, *or about 1%* of the combined Medicare-Medicaid budgets, is spent on home health care. Furthermore, it was pointed out that unrealistic regulations allowed people to receive care in hospitals or from medical personnel but not from competent people in the home. Most health insurance is geared to crisis care, hospital stays, and physician-prescribed drugs or therapies rather than prevention, self-help, and home care.

Despite hardship and disincentives, most families have struggled to raise their children without recourse to institutional settings. Collectively they have received about 5% of the total resources, whereas the 5% who have been institutionalized have received the lion's share, approximately 95% of the available money and resources. Thus, it is inevitable that large facilities are criticized on the basis of cost alone, although clearly cost is not the only issue.

Unfortunately, the legal suits that first recognized a disabled person's right to treatment, to freedom from harm, and to the least restrictive setting were brought on behalf of those already in institutions. Court orders that require the upgrading of institutions, the extensive hiring of additional staff, and millions of dollars in legal fees have meant that the institutionalized population has received advocacy at the expense of those struggling, sometimes desperately, to remain in the community. The following account resembles more than one person's struggle.

A father left his wife and son when the boy was 3 years old. The husband was not prepared to deal with the son's disabilities. The mother received welfare until she was able to find employment. Alone, for years, she daily carried her son in braces to a babysitter in order to work.

When the son had grown the mother found a new companion who was willing to marry her provided she found a place to put her son. The new husband was also not prepared to handle her son with a disability. There were advantages, she felt, to her son as well, if he moved. He would benefit from being in an environment with people his own age, and with assistance from someone more capable than she, he could get to community functions. But she couldn't find any facility near her that would accept him. The admissions at the state facility were closed to her because the state said he had to stay in the community, and the group home two blocks from her home was accepting people from hundreds of miles away, but wouldn't accept her son because he had not lived in a state facility.

This woman's predicament is not uncommon now that institutions are under mandate to reduce their populations in order to comply with constitutional requirements for least restrictive settings. Furthermore, they are struggling to meet the medically oriented accreditation standards. In order to obtain federal money for their clients, institutions have to meet guidelines that are costing millions in renovations. This adds up to a double bind for people in the community.

A dangerous result of the mandated deinstitutionalization has been the dumping of people into the community without proper supports for successful living. This gives supporters of normalization and other modern philosophies a setback in community development and support. People protest that community living cannot work. Many of the people dumped into the community have ended up brutalized and dead. Others have faced reinstitutionalization for lack of an alternative.

Probably one of the most unfortunate consequences of spending so much money inappropriately has been the polarization between parents and other advocates. The haves are against the have-nots, with no one feeling very happy or confident for the future. Parents and professional staff have historically been at opposite ends, but never so drastically as now, when it is crucial that they unite. Parents, traditionally the advocates for their children, have been considered overly emotional and guilt ridden, and unable to make rational decisions without the assistance of a professional. Medical professionals, in their zeal to advise parents in the best way, have mistakenly been under the impression that they have all the answers. Hence, we have a profession that is still making recommendations to place disabled children under institutional care.

Professional decision makers are responsible for the greater percentage of state funds going to state facilities while the greater percentage of disabled people live in the communities. They are also responsible for the lack of faith in community services among parents of institutionalized children.

## NEW DIRECTIONS

The alternatives to institutions and other inappropriate residential services are many. Some states are adopting plans for residential continua and individualized placements. Four exemplary models are described in this book. Parents and families should become very familiar with these alternatives so that they can seek out the best care for their offspring, so they can be articulate and knowledgeable in their lobbying, and so that they have their own peace of mind, knowing that services are improving, however slowly.

A growing number of court cases sanction our efforts to provide community services. In *Morales* v. *Turman* (11), a federal court went to the heart of the problem:

> The state may not circumvent the Constitution by simply refusing to create any alternatives to incarceration; it must act affirmatively to foster such alternatives as now exist only in rudimentary form, and to build new programs suited to the needs of hundreds of its children that do not need institutional care.

In the widely publicized Willowbrook case, the defendants sought to define "least restrictive setting" as whatever was presently available even if it was simply a newer, more modern institution. The parents went back into court again and again. Finally the judge made it clear that the needs of the individual from the individual's perspective and not the needs and convenience of the service providers were to be the deciding factor. The court ordered a plan to create appropriate community settings.

R. J. Broderick, the judge in the Pennhurst case in Pennsylvania, recently made a revolutionary decision. He ruled that the contemporary lack of community alternatives was no reason to place anyone in an institution. He mandated that proper settings must be created and that institutionalization is unconstitutional—a milestone for freedom!

With recognition in the law, public education, and parent and professional unity, our dream for the future can be realized. And in that dream we see many things.

We see that fully subsidized adoptions must be available to families who qualilfy. Medicaid and other supports must be guaranteed, if needed for expenses beyond the cost of typical child-rearing. Foster and family care must be supported at levels that do not penalize families for making commitments to children with need for complex or specialized care. Present restrictions under Medicaid and Crippled Children's Services often force families to travel to out-of-town clinics and purchase certain equipment at their own expense.

We see homes for children that will approximate a family as nearly as possible in size and living arrangements. Group homes for adults will not run on a houseparent or family model but rather on a basis of people sharing their lives as equals. The state will provide significant funding for community residential programs, and whenever federal, state, or local dollars are used for housing, a portion of the housing shall be accessible to people who are disabled.

Those agencies common to all citizens will be encouraged to develop specialized services and to share staff with specialty organizations in order to develop this expertise. For example, some adult education programs at junior colleges are beginning to offer courses that disabled people want, such as driver's education. If a person has experience with hand controls, that person could be hired as a consultant or teacher with the school's program rather than holding the course at a segregated facility for the disabled.

Medical standards as a prerequisite for federal dollars should be challenged. Often they increase costs significantly and do not result in better care. Regulations must be changed to emphasize prevention, self-help, and home care. Funding sources should be made available for these purposes.

The disabled person or his or her family must be allowed to choose those individuals who will provide attendant services and who will have access to their homes and bodies. No third party checks shall be allowed. The person must be able to hire, fire, and pay his or her own help in order to hold them accountable. Horror stories abound when agencies disregard input from the disabled persons.

Furthermore, payment by an agency perpetuates a form of bondage in which a person is not free to make intimate decisions about his or her own body. It also violates equal protection as compared to others, such as recipients of welfare funds, who, being duly qualified, are free to use the money as they see fit. "Vendorization" of services is one of the hottest issues today and will need to be resolved in the courts.

Residential settings should belong to or be rented by disabled people in every case possible. If funding is sufficient for someone else to buy a facility out of operating expenses, then disabled people, too, ought to be able to build equity just as do other people.

Coordinating agencies must ensure that disabled people can move from town to town and state to state just as their families do, without losing services. Community specialists must be available to help families obtain the kinds of service and funding that are immediately secured once the government takes custody.

The new wave of human service professionals who are fighting for community residential programs often are doing so without knowledge of the powerful resource they have in families. By families, we mean natural parents, adoptive and foster parents, and siblings. Too frequently it is assumed that families who have institutionalized their children or families who have kept their children home well into adulthood are overprotective and against greater independence. Although this is perhaps often true at a certain level, it is also true that parents are receptive to education. They need to be involved in the movement so that they can learn to support modern philosophy and contribute in their own way to their children's well-being. Inevitably, parents have the power to make the demands. Without solidarity, parents and professionals may be casualties in the entire movement toward better services.

We have tried to present the issues we think are critical to parents and families today. They are the heart of improved services for tomorrow. Yesterday's beliefs, unless attacked head on, will crush our spirit. Among these principles for the future will be improved attitudes and treatment of families with disabled members. More services and funds will be given to natural families. Due process of law will be followed and agencies recommending removal of a child from his home must show that reasonable support services, such as counseling, training, respite, and homemaking help, have been tried. In tomorrow lies the alternative beyond the institution and the sanctity of liberty.

## REFERENCES

1. *Olmstead* v. *U.S.* 1928. U.S. Supreme Court Reports 277:438.
2. Reader responses. 1977. The Exceptional Parent, August, p. 56.
3. Case history: Deinstitutionalization. 1977. The Exceptional Parent, December, pp. 21–24.
4. Wolfensberger, W., and Glenn, L. 1975. Program Analysis of Service Systems. National Institute on Mental Retardation, Toronto.
5. Santiestevan, H. 1975. Deinstitutionalization: Out of Their Beds and into the Streets. American Federation of State, County, and Municipal Employees, Washington, D.C.
6. Stockdale, L. 1976. A legal advocate's experience. Amicus, December, pp. 29–30.
7. Wellette, R. 1977. Letter to the editor. Schenectady Gazette, January 11.
8. Letter to the editor. 1977. Playboy, May.
9. Veile, L. 1976. Is anybody watching? Reader's Digest, March, pp. 114–118.
10. DDO Newsletter. 1977. March/April.
11. *Morales* v. *Turman.* U.S. Supreme Court Reports.

# ENCOR AND BEYOND

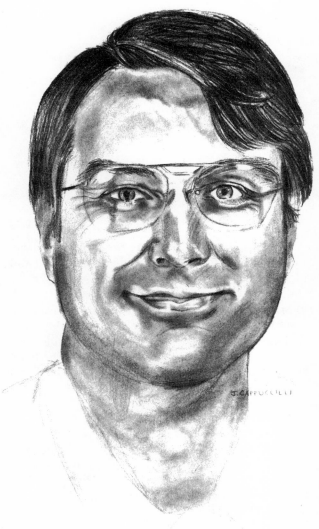

Wade Hitzing

*I* *work at the Center for the Development of* Community Alternative Service Systems (CASS), located at the Medical Center of the University of Nebraska. It is affiliated with the Meyer Children's Rehabilitation Institute. CASS exists to provide technical assistance and training so that "developmentally disabled" citizens will have the same residential, vocational, educational, and social opportunities available to all other citizens. It provides program and manpower development assistance throughout Federal Region VII: Nebraska, Kansas, Missouri, and Iowa. CASS works with community-based service programs, community colleges, and universities to help establish broad-based training networks.

CASS employs four community service specialists. They assist the community programs in our region to develop high quality integrative services for developmentally disabled citizens. Our services range from assisting a State Planning Council in preparing its annual plan to going to Sioux City, Iowa and testifying before a zoning board for a residence whose opening is blocked by an objecting church. CASS does not offer direct services. We suggest how things ought to be, help write out service plans, and then drive back in our air-conditioned Medical Center car, leaving the service and advocacy groups with the difficult job of actually implementing the plan.

I had the good fortune to serve as the Director of the Division of Program Development and Training for the Eastern Nebraska Community Office of Retardation (ENCOR) for 1 year during 1975 and 1976. Many of my comments in this chapter focus on lessons I learned from observing ENCOR's experience in community program development, especially in the area of residential services.[1]

## THE ENCOR SYSTEM

### State Organization

An overview of the ENCOR model is provided in this section. The organizational structure for Nebraska's services for persons labeled "mentally retarded" is shown in Figure 1. The Department of Public Institutions administers Nebraska's one state institution (recently labeled the Beatrice State Developmental Center) and the Office of Mental Retardation, the state regulatory agency for community mental retardation programs.

Nebraska's community service system is divided into six regional programs. ENCOR is located in the eastern part of the state, Region VI. This region includes only about 3% of the state's total area. However, approximately 35% of the state's population, 1.5 million people, resides in ENCOR's service area. Enormous demographic differences exist among the five counties included in ENCOR's area. It encompasses urban Omaha, which is fairly typical of any relatively large city, and areas in outlying counties that are very rural. The total case load for ENCOR during the period 1976–1977 was 541 adults and 350 children. Table 1 summarizes the number of clients who received services purchased or provided by ENCOR.

### ENCOR's Organization

The administrative structure of ENCOR can be seen in Figure 2. A commissioner is selected by each of the five county boards comprising ENCOR's service region to be on the governing board for an

---

[1]Ed Skarnulis was Director of Residential Services at this time and provided much of the information in this chapter.

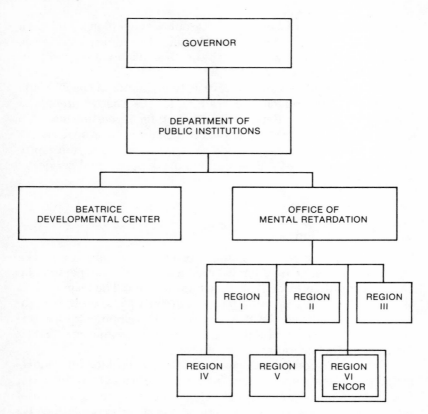

**Figure 1.** Nebraska's service structure for the "mentally retarded."

**Table 1.** Number of children and adults receiving ENCOR services in fiscal 1976–1977

| Service type | Children | Adults | Total[a] |
|---|---|---|---|
| Residential | 102 | 149 | 251 |
| Educational | 146 | 4 | 150 |
| Guidance | 350 | 541 | 891 |
| Specialized | 176 | 176 | 352 |
| Transportation | 99 | 165 | 264 |
| Recreation | 0 | 0 | 0 |
| Motor development | 149 | 99 | 248 |
| Vocational | 3 | 315 | 318 |

[a]Duplicated counts of clients in every service they received throughout the year.

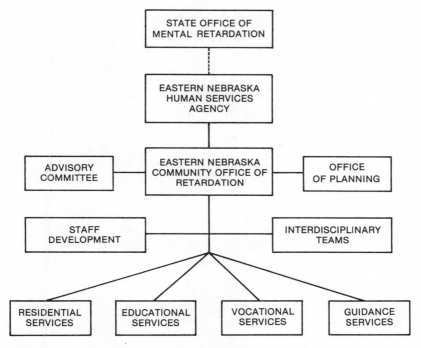

**Figure 2.** Organizational structure of ENCOR's regional community program.

umbrella agency, the Eastern Nebraska Human Service Agency (ENHSA). ENHSA includes the Office of Aging, Office of Retardation, and Office of Mental Health. The members of the ENHSA governing board set administrative policy and approve major decisions. The director of ENHSA has administrative responsibility over the ENCOR director. ENCOR is suborganized into residential, educational, vocational, and guidance service divisions. The other functions shown provide support to these divisions.

## ENCOR'S RESIDENTIAL SERVICES

### Overall Organization

The organizational format for ENCOR's Residential Services is illustrated in Figure 3. The personnel who operate this system include one division director and four area coordinators. Each coor-

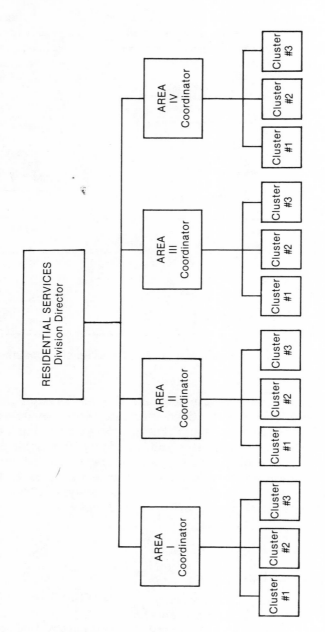

**Figure 3.** Organizational structure of ENCOR's residential services.

dinator is responsible for a number of geographically dispersed clusters. A cluster consists of a core training residence, serving usually three to six clients, and an array of individualized placements (alternative living units), which spin off each core residence. The staff for each cluster includes a manager, who primarily works out of the training residence, an assistant manager of the core residence, an assistant manager of dispersed services, and line staff. The assistant manager in charge of dispersed services has primary responsibility for supervising and providing support to the alternative living units organized by the cluster: apartments, condominiums, independent living arrangements, and foster homes. Line staff are called "residential assistants," a title that has changed many times during ENCOR's history.

One factor that differentiates ENCOR's programs from those operated in other areas of the country is that ENCOR is a monolithic system. ENCOR doesn't contract with private residential vendors. The staff person who goes out to a client's apartment once a week and the staff member who works 40 hours a week in a training residence are both employees of ENCOR. Foster parents are also ENCOR employees.

## Core Training Residences

ENCOR's core training residences range from large group homes with capacities of up to eight residents to small houses with three clients. People with disabilities come to core residences as a transition to more independent, individualized community placements. Core residence staff recruit, train, and draw up contracts with community members who are interested in providing community residential placements. Community members are recruited by newspaper advertising, notices posted at universities, United Way, radio and television advertising, and church announcements.

Each training residence serves as a central "back-up" and support mechanism for all of its individualized placement settings. Residential assistants go out from core residences to provide support for alternative living unit staff, and core training residences, along with contracted community homes, serve as temporary back-up placements when crises occur.

## Alternative Living Units

The design of alternative living units ranges from live-in staff in an apartment with one or two clients to off-site staff support for individual clients on a daily, weekly, or monthly basis. No two alternative living units are exactly alike. One of the more famous ENCOR alternative living arrangements is the Developmental Maximation Unit, located at the County Hospital, which serves multiply handicapped, medically fragile children. Most children are placed in nontraditional foster care settings, which may overcome many of the difficulties of typical foster care. Foster parents are provided with adequate training, and are contracted with to provide clearly defined services. The point is to try to employ indigenous community homes as placement sites and community members as program staff because doing this results in a more normalized approach to human management.

With no mandatory staffing patterns, salaries, regulations, fire codes, or architecture, you can't find an alternative living unit unless you know where to look. ENCOR has found that communities are filled with people who are able to share and teach. With adequate pre-screening, continuing training and supports, and decent wages, people can be mobilized to use their own homes and apartments to offer high quality, integrated services and individualized, in-home training. The alternative living unit model works because people in natural communities can develop skills to support handicapped people in their progress toward more independent living.

### In-Home Services

ENCOR's residential division also offers in-home services to natural families that range from babysitting to direct work with parents on changing a problem behavior, to crisis in-home support. ENCOR operates on the policy that no external residential service can duplicate a young person's healthy family system. The bond between a person and his or her family weakens when they are separated by distance, for long periods, or if they have to live with large numbers of unrelated persons. Supporting the family early is important. Parents are encouraged to identify their needs for relief periods, counseling and support, in-home training, short-term crisis assistance, or special appliances in the home. With adult clients, the important issue is to support the family's efforts to help the client achieve independent living. ENCOR helps parents to assist their adult handicapped offspring plan for a job, find a home, and live as normal and as independent a life as possible.

ENCOR has found that it is less expensive and more effective to support natural homes with a wide range of backup services than to remove people from their homes and serve them elsewhere. When a decision is made that a child or adult must leave home in spite of all supportive attempts, every effort is put into finding a community placement close to home. ENCOR staffs work to find as integrated a setting as possible with the shortest length of stay possible. If the move must be permanent, great care is taken to avoid placing the person into an institution. The important thing is to find an alternative residence that supports the fullest development for the person in the most integrated setting possible.

## Staff-Client Ratio and Costs

The staff-client ratio in ENCOR's residential settings varies tremendously depending on the nature of the service being delivered. Five or six full-time staff members, for example, may operate a group home for three children with severe behavior problems whereas one part-time staff member may serve as a supervisor/visitor for 6 to 10 semi-independent clients. Client costs also vary widely but are relatively easy to relate to each client because of the *individual placement* approach. Fees for services range from $100 per day at the Developmental Maximation Unit to $20–$30 per day in core training residences, to $10–$40 per day in alternative living units, to $0.50 per day for periodic in-home services (these are best estimates possible as of December, 1977).

## BASIC RESIDENTIAL SERVICE ISSUES

ENCOR's experience in community service development offers a number of important lessons for those interested in developing alternatives to institutions. First, the history of ENCOR underscores the relative importance of philosophy versus technology in achieving advances in service development. Second, the experience of ENCOR, and other advanced, community-based systems, advises against developing a permanent, facility-based service continuum. More flexible service systems are needed. Third, ENCOR has learned that high quality residential services must be designed and delivered on an individual basis. Finally, ENCOR's experience strongly suggests that we should begin by developing the most integrated aspects of service systems and only develop specialized services when absolutely necessary.

## Philosophy versus Technology

We've found that one of the major stumbling blocks to community service development is a lack of understanding or commitment to appropriate program philosophy. For example, when Federal Judge O. Judd in the Willowbrook case was asked why so many "retarded" citizens live in Willowbrook, he had a simple answer: "There's no other alternative!" The fact that no other alternatives existed in the state of New York at that time had nothing to do with the technology of human services, nor had it anything to do with knowledge of how to run residential programs. Rather, it had to do with the basic values and program philosophy of the service system.

About 10 years ago I was involved in a behavior modification program at Kazamazoo State Hospital. I thought that if the hospital could reduce its population by 30% during the 2 years I was there, it was going to be due to the efforts of our behavior modification program. It surely wasn't! The population was reduced by 30%, but it was reduced because the department simply adopted a new philosophy of residential service. The new philosophy said, "We're not going to do this any more; large congregate institutions are not viable service units. We're moving away from them." This change took place because key decision makers changed their *basic program philosophy.*

I don't know of a single situation in which system changes were primarily motivated by technology. Sound teaching technology does have to be available in order to integrate children with special needs into normal school programs. Technology provides means and procedures, but it does not provide goals and objectives. You have to be able to change behavior, but simply knowing how to change behavior is not sufficient in itself. The development of quality programs depends on a guiding philosophy and a commitment to implement it. In ENCOR's case this philosophical perspective encompasses three basic components: 1) assurance of legal and human rights, 2) adherence to the developmental model of growth and development, and 3) actualization of the principle of normalization in human services.

It is very important to use philosophy as a guidepost when devising program technology. When I first arrived at ENCOR we asked our vocational programs to evaluate their services. Service providers knew lots about outcome data; they were already plotting various indices of clients' behavior. Radical behaviorist consultants had six-cycle charts pasted all over their walls and were selling wrist counters. These service providers knew outcome, but often there was little emphasis on how to get there, and little recognition that the nature of the means is just as important as the objectives being sought. ENCOR has achieved major changes in this area. These changes are reflected in the agency's policies and in the ways behavior management procedures are applied. ENCOR has allowed basic program philosophy to influence technology as much as possible rather than vice versa. Some of the evaluation questions that we are beginning to ask ourselves in this area are included in Figures 4 and 5. If a 35-year-old adult is being given M & M's as reinforcers at 2:00 p.m. in a sheltered workshop setting in order to learn how to put on his pants, you've got some serious questions to ask—even if he learns how to put on his pants.

A recent personal experience reinforced how important philosophical considerations are in developing sound service programs. I served on a task force to plan a residential program for 12 children with severe disabilities. These children were going to school 5 days a week at the Medical Center in Omaha. Their residential program had been operated in keeping with the medical model at one time, but had been recently changed to a group home approach. The children weren't moved from the Medical Center. Instead, one large "group home" was set up on their ward. The task force agreed that we wanted to move away from this "group home" approach and that individual placements based on individual needs were in order. As we started reviewing all of the children's needs, however, I soon realized that we easily could have ended up moving them all to Beatrice Developmental Center. That's right—by carefully listing all the children's needs and the ways to meet them, we could have ended up moving them all to a state institution. Fortunately, the members of the task force were committed to certain fundamental principles of service development that dictated an alternative course of action. The program that we designed calls for individual placements in foster homes.

## Problems with a Continuum Approach

The overwhelming acceptance of the "continuum of services" concept is proving to be a problem. States and communities are saying, "We must develop a continuum of services in order to meet all the needs of our handicapped citizens." These continua are almost invariably organized around different environments like those

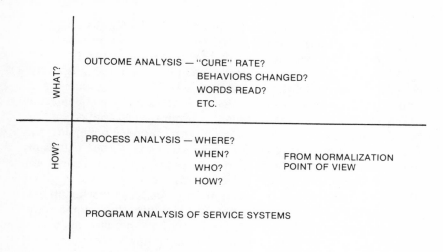

**Figure 4.** Program evaluation considerations based on behavioral technology and the principles of normalization.

depicted in Figure 6. The notion is that since a geographical area has $X$ number of profoundly, severely, and moderately disabled citizens, you need $Y$ number of work activity centers and $Z$ number of sheltered workshops. This logic makes it very easy to develop a state plan.

The development of a residential continuum generally has advantages over the previous alternatives: institutions and supported natural homes. I see serious problems emerging in community development, however, if we continue to focus on developing service continua composed largely of specialized facilities that place people in different living environments on the basis of certain labels or classifications. Some day we will be faced with

| REINFORCEMENT RELATED | NORMALIZATION RELATED |
|---|---|
| 1. EFFECTIVE REINFORCER? | 1. AGE APPROPRIATE? |
| 2. IMMEDIACY? | 2. PHYSICAL CONTEXT? |
| 3. FREQUENCY? | 3. TIME OF DAY? |
| 4. SCHEDULE? | 4. DEVIANCY JUXTAPOSITION? |

**Figure 5.** Evaluative criteria based on behavioral technology and the principle of normalization.

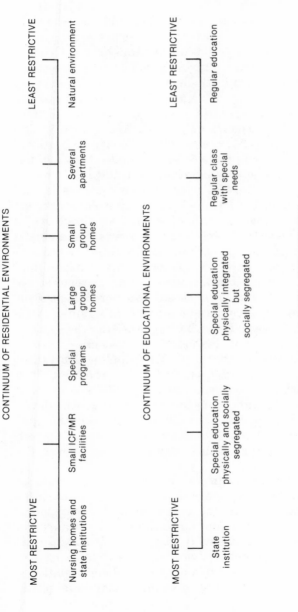
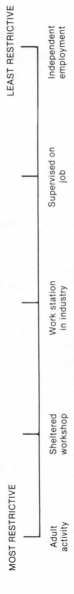

CONTINUUM OF RESIDENTIAL ENVIRONMENTS

MOST RESTRICTIVE | LEAST RESTRICTIVE

Nursing homes and state institutions — Small ICF/MR facilities — Special programs — Large group homes — Small group homes — Several apartments — Natural environment

CONTINUUM OF EDUCATIONAL ENVIRONMENTS

MOST RESTRICTIVE | LEAST RESTRICTIVE

State institution — Special education physically and socially segregated — Special education physically integrated but socially segregated — Regular class with special needs — Regular education

CONTINUUM OF VOCATIONAL ENVIRONMENTS

MOST RESTRICTIVE | LEAST RESTRICTIVE

Adult activity — Sheltered workshop — Work station in industry — Supervised on job — Independent employment

**Figure 6.** Typical service continua of residential, educational, and vocational environments.

changing these facilities and doing so may not be easy. For example, in a small town in Iowa $600,000 were invested in building a new addition to the county care facility. The addition was to be used, supposedly, to meet the vocational needs of the people who lived in the facility. Later, a proposal was brought to the county commissioners to fund a more physically and socially integrated vocational training program in the downtown area. The county commissioners said, "Two years ago you convinced us to put $600,000 into the county care facility and now you want $6,000 a year to rent something else. We built you a fine facility 5 miles outside of town. Go there." So now all of the city's vocational training programs are going to be 5 miles outside of town, a further barrier to the vocational integration of disabled citizens.

Another negative feature of most service continua is that they place a tremendous burden on *clients* for movement. For example, one state plan I read recently used the word "graduate" a number of times, always in quotes. The notion was that a person moved into the residential system initially by being placed in a nursing home or large group home. Once clients "shaped up," they "graduated" to a smaller group home. If they learned certain skills in the group home, they "graduated" to a more independent placement unit. The very existence of such a continuum of facilities forces the client to earn his or her way through the system. The underlying philosophy of this model is not at all consistent with civil rights decisions in other areas. The Supreme Court ruled in the 1960s that Black people had a right to ride in the front of the bus and to go to their neighborhood schools, rights based simply on their citizenship—not rights they had to earn. But with "developmentally disabled" people we have said you must *earn* the right to live in an integrated setting. You must behave yourself before we'll ever give you this right. This is clearly a basic form of discrimination.

Another reason for caution in our rush to develop service continua is that good services change over time in response to shifts in client population and in response to societal needs and opportunities. One critical factor contributing to the success of ENCOR is that its service system is designed to be flexible. It adopts residential models that reflect newer, more progressive thinking. EN-COR's residential services were originally set up along a relatively traditional group home model. The core cluster-individual place-

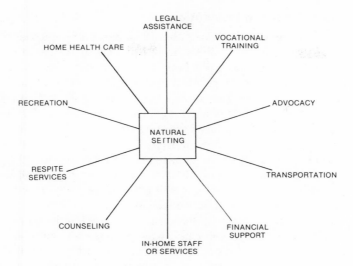

**Figure 7.** Community-based services needed by some adults with special needs.

ment concept was adopted to allow more individualized, integrated modes of service. There has been movement from reliance on a "couple" houseparent role to a more professional staff approach, and the introduction of a more complex geographical regionalization-cluster approach to system management. The system also now serves more severely handicapped clients than in its early years.

ENCOR is beginning to meet clients' needs by doing away with the continuum. Maybe a continuum is necessary to meet your needs at some point in time for development, staff, and funding. Instead of saying that we must have eight different kinds of living places for handicapped people, however, try to have each person live in the most natural setting possible. For a child this means the natural family or at least a foster home; for adults it means living by themselves, with other adults, or whatever arrangement they choose. Many adults need supportive residential services. There must be 50 or so supportive services that adults with disabilities might need at one time or another in order to maintain a chosen living arrangement. Some of the more important of these services are outlined in Figure 7.

## Individualization and Integration

All residential service decisions should be based on analyses of: 1) basic program philosophy, 2) the individual client's strengths and needs, and 3) the available placement and support options. There are tremendous implications for a residential system if you don't assume that everybody needs out-of-home services. It has implications for questions like when the service is provided, what type, whom it is provided for, and where the service is provided. For example, if a child needs a program because he or she roams at night, disturbs the neighborhood, or causes other problems that the parents can't handle, then the residential service must be provided in the home. The family's problems will never be solved by replacing the home. Ed Skarnulis (ENCOR Residential Director) told me about the case of a child who lived in an ENCOR residential placement 5 days a week and went home each weekend. Somebody finally asked why the child couldn't live at home all the time. They learned that the only reason the child was in an out-of-home program was that his mother had a job as a bartender and could not be at home from 3:00 p.m. to 11:00 p.m. Because she could not afford a babysitter her child was forced to live 5 days a week in a group home. Arrangements were made for babysitting services and the child moved out of the expensive, specialized residence back into his natural home.

Analyzing the reasons people are moving into your residential programs can tremendously influence your service program. If a child or adult is in your program because of a problem in the home, then this consideration should affect your service. You can implement a thousand behavior management programs for a person without making any impact on the reasons that person moved out of the natural home. Moreover, the person may stay in your program forever because you are not attacking the real reason for initial placement. People often automatically assume that it is acceptable practice to supply residential services simply because a person is labeled "severely handicapped" or "behavior disordered." Residential services are rarely questioned as long as the client has a label. But my observations of the ENCOR program have convinced me that the real reasons for placement are related to the *needs of individual clients* and to the *needs of their families*. Children with histories of not being toilet trained for 5 years are suddenly referred for out-of-home placement. Why after 5 years are parents now seeking residential services? It probably has something to do with their current status: a divorce, illness, or additional children. The real problem is generally the lack of supportive services available in the family's community. Every case must receive individual consideration.

## Planning Issues

Let's reflect for a few moments on what is happening in the area of social integration. I firmly believe that the war between institutions and community programs has been won. If I were going to invest my money in Nebraska so that I could buy a car next year, I might invest it in the Beatrice State Developmental Center, because Beatrice is still going very strong. But if I wanted to invest my money to retire, I would not invest it in Beatrice. The strong anti-segregated institution stance of Section 504 of the Rehabilitation Act of 1973 and the recent outcome of the Pennhurst case signal the long-term demise of state institutions. Section 504 maintains that all programs that receive federal money, benefit from federal service, or utilize federal property must serve handicapped citizens in the most integrated settings possible. It forces the service program to demonstrate that segregated services are necessary to meet the client's needs. The Pennhurst decision states that it is illegal to provide services to mentally retarded citizens in institutions like Pennhurst State Hospital and mandates shutting down this large facility.

I'm pleased by the decline of the institutions, but I'm concerned that we are not developing fully integrated community alternatives to take their place. It is important to begin planning and development of truly integrated service programs. We might do well to make the naïve assumption that every disabled adult who comes from our service area can live in the community and can work in some business or industry or go to school with nondisabled classmates. If we start there and it later becomes necessary to compromise and use some segregated programs, we'll know that the compromise is really based on the system's needs and not on the client's needs. For example, we may have to meet a specific child's needs by placing the child in a special training home. But we must recognize the reason(s) for this compromise, i.e., the fact that this is the only program available right now, this is the only kind of funding we can get, the parents are fighting us, or our community staff isn't adequately trained. The worst thing that I see in communities is that often such compromises are rationalized as being based on *client needs*. This approach removes any motivation to ever change things. If most programs really adhered to their mission statements, in which they say they don't serve people who could be served in less restrictive settings, they wouldn't serve very many people.

Along with many others, I have been involved for a number of years in developing community alternatives to institutions, and I have been proud to be involved in this work. Co-workers and I sometimes sit around and pat each other on the back. "We are developing alternatives to institutions; aren't we good people?" Many of the people we serve have had to live in 2,000- and 3,000-bed institutions, but now we are developing group homes in their home communities. That's fine. However, another way of looking at these same community programs, which ENCOR has begun to realize, is that specialized programs, whether group homes or sheltered workshops, really serve as alternatives to existing, more integrated, generic programs. They may be more integrative than large institutions but they are still different than those available to all other citizens. We must strive to provide only those specialized services that handicapped individuals cannot get through utilizing generic services.

An analogy may be drawn between providing residential services to people with severe disabilities and attempting to make a regular hospital a nice place to stay. You'd have at least two vastly different ways of doing it available to you. One would be to take the hospital as it currently exists, bring in some architects, service providers, consumers, and look at the hospital and say, "Let's make it nice." You'd bring in potted plants, paintings, but you still wouldn't have a place where you or I would like to spend 5 days of our life. We could do something else, however. We could renovate the downtown Hilton Hotel. It doesn't have any surgery rooms or any sterile rooms so we would have to construct them. We wouldn't construct more of these rooms than we need, however, and I think we could end up with a place where we would like to stay. There is one hospital like this in Connecticut, and people wait in line to go there.

The long-term dangers of developing facility-based service continua are tremendous. We talk about skyrocketing institutional costs, but look at the costs of developing an extensive residential continuum. Find or construct a building, buy or lease it, furnish it, place clients, and assign staff members. By the time you get to the most integrated end of the continuum, the least restrictive segment, there are no money, staff, or clients. All the clients have been placed in group homes and the group homes cannot operate with fewer people. The outcome you frequently see in residential and vocational programs is a lack of staff for placement and follow-up when a client moves to an apartment or gets a job—almost all of the staff is used to run the segregated programs.

Although you necessarily may have some segregated programs at first due to funding constraints, eventually more integrated alternatives must be built. If the segregated programs remain on the continuum, people will be placed there, there's no doubt about it.

Clearly, the existence of already segregated community programs is going to be a barrier to the development of integrated service systems. In some states the barrier is lack of funds, but in most states it's that the wrong funds are available (i.e., Title XIX). In our region we still have the problem of existing laws and regulations as barriers. Because of Title XIX funding parameters, more beds and cottages on the grounds of institutions are under construction. Many states have reached the ceiling of their Title XIX monies and community programs are being cut back rather than expanded. The issue is not that we don't have the needed resources; it's a matter of where we are putting our resources. A number of states are going to make strong moves toward using Title XIX to establish highly integrated community programs. Our reading of the rules and regulations says nothing about not being able to use Title XIX funds to start integrated programs; the barrier is simply existing federal, regional, and state interpretations.

## STAFF DEVELOPMENT

One important thing to understand is that although ENCOR has been viewed as providing exemplary residential service, it has never had an outstanding training program. In fact, I don't know of any community-based program in the United States that does. If there is one aspect of community service development of which we should be ashamed, it is training. The state hospital that I worked for in Kalamazoo may not have always trained people to do the right things, but they surely had a serious commitment of money, time, and people toward training.

The training personnel for ENCOR's staff development programs currently include one director and three trainers. Staff training begins with an orientation to the ENCOR system. This orientation covers system relationships; the history of attitudes toward and services for the "mentally retarded"; and other areas, such as human and legal rights, behavior management, precision teaching, normalization, and individual program plan development. This orientation is followed within 3 months by a 1-day session of normalization and PASS. Additionally, during the course of their first year, ENCOR employees attend 1-day training sessions on behavior management, writing behavioral objectives, and individual program planning. Most information is transmitted via lecture. A few slide shows, videotapes, and movies are used. Written handouts are supplied to supplement lecture content.

ENCOR, like most service programs, operates on the assumption that if you've received $X$ hours of instruction, you're trained for something. There are obvious weaknesses associated with neglect of competency-based instruction. The unique thing about ENCOR, however, the thing that has always impressed me about the system, is its tremendous commitment to philosophy, both in its training and its service programs. I think that the widespread philosophical commitment on the part of ENCOR's staff is partly attributable to its training program but more to the fact that its leadership mandates and models a strong commitment to "normalization."

Before coming to ENCOR I worked in Michigan trying to train hospital staff in behavior management. My dream was to go into a community agency or a hospital and teach staff members to talk about shaping, fading, and schedules of reinforcement to such a degree that it permeated their whole existence. But this strategy totally failed to make meaningful improvements in clients' lives. When I came to the ENCOR program I was hit right in the face— they had done it! They were helping clients achieve more independent and productive lives primarily because of a radical commitment to a philosophy—normalization. I think this approach may be easier. You first need to get the staff excited about what ought to be (philosophy) before you can talk about how to achieve it (technology).

The biggest reason for staff turnover may be that people don't understand what they're getting into. One important aspect of training for ENCOR's residential staff is an early session where staff members talk about what it is like to be a residential assistant and what it is like to be a residential manager. ENCOR has learned to be honest early about what new staff people are getting into, and this has helped reduce staff turnover later.

One of the key factors in deinstitutionalizing the service systems may lie in learning to deinstitutionalize training. Once, while I was writing a paper on this topic, I began making writing mistakes. The mistakes I made involved substituting *service words* for *training words* because the fundamental issues are the same. If you live in western Nebraska and you want to be trained to work with disabled citizens, you have to move away from your home community. You have to fit into an existing career preparation system. They don't write individual program plans for you. We must develop deinstitutionalized strategies for training staffs just as we must develop similar strategies for serving clients. Heavy emphasis should be placed on field-based training; i.e., on delivering training in real community service contexts. Decades of research on transfer of training indicate that maximum generalization occurs when training is delivered in real versus classroom settings or simulated settings.

Finally, the two major problems I see with respect to training residential service staffs are appropriate or nonexistent curricula and insufficient application of good educational technology. Curriculum materials are not available in many areas and what does exist is often inappropriate ideologically or technologically. If you know of a film on epilepsy that presents technically correct information and shows clients in normal settings without a medical model, "sickness" approach, let me know. I don't know of any. Much work is needed in the areas of curriculum development and instructional technology, particularly with respect to serving "severely handicapped" citizens. I recommend the staff training materials recently developed in California known as *Way To Go* (1).

## CONCLUSION

This chapter has centered on the structure of the ENCOR service system and on lessons to be learned from ENCOR's experience. I have attempted to emphasize: 1) the relative importance of basic program philosophy over technology in service development, 2) that it is a serious mistake to develop a continuum of different residential environments, 3) that services are best designed for and delivered to clients, and 4) that flexible, *specialized* services should be developed only when all attempts to utilize generic services have failed. The future of community-based residential services seems very bright. It will be all the brighter if we can learn from each other—from our failures and successes.

## QUESTIONS AND ANSWERS

QUESTION: What sort of parent cooperation and involvement does ENCOR receive to convince resistive parents to move their sons and daughters out of institutions?

HITZING: As you may be aware, ENCOR was begun by the Greater Omaha Association for Retarded Citizens. ENCOR was eventually spun off from this parent group as it got bigger. Parent confidence in ENCOR's programs is very strong. Parents are probably the strongest force in getting other parents involved in the program and in overcoming initial resistance.

QUESTION: Most of your efforts are with clients who have special needs associated with mental retardation. My agency serves clients who manifest other handicaps, such as autism. Can one service program serve all clients?

HITZING: Categorical programs don't seem to be necessary. A large number of clients in the ENCOR system have other disabilities. If you were diagnostically precise about it, the primary disabling condition of many ENCOR clients would be autism or some other categorical distinction. These clients are served, however, because ENCOR tries to provide as individualized a service as possible. I don't see why you would need to have a separate residential program for people called "autistic" or "epileptic." They may have special needs, but that doesn't mean you have to establish a totally separate program.

We recently designed a model, 5-day-a-week residential program for children. Three of them are diagnosed "autistic." The particular environments that we developed for each of these three children were somewhat different than they would have been for deaf-blind children or retarded children, but the same system served all of them.

One point that I failed to make earlier is that I'm convinced you can serve everybody with the same service system but not with the same service program. One residential system can handle everyone's needs because if you employ an individual placement approach you end up with different programs for each client. The notion that you would set up different service systems with different funding mechanisms goes counter to everything ENCOR and CASS are trying to work toward. I think you must do a good job of convincing parents that you are sensitive to their child's disability and that you're going to meet their specific needs.

Question: Have there been any tools devised that can measure how well persons who have been institutionalized have changed in their perception of themselves after moving to an integrated setting?

HITZING: There are very few, if any, data even on behavior change from institutions to community settings. I think everybody here who has experience with deinstitutionalization, however, has a gut-level feeling about the positive behavioral and attitudinal changes we see as clients become a part of the community. The data to answer your question are sorely needed.

QUESTION: Has there been resistance to moving half a dozen handicapped people into one area?

HITZING: I think one prejudice we have when we hear somebody talk about really integrated settings, with emphasis on individual placements, is that such an approach is very radical. And we often equate being radical with being difficult to pull off. In truth, it's a lot easier to place people—logistically, financially, and every other way—in much more integrated settings. I once attended a symposium on normalization. The moderator of the symposium very angrily read an article from an Indianapolis newspaper, which said that a zoning board had voted down a 12-bed group home. She was incensed. She said, "It's 1977 and they're still prejudiced." But I had some sympathy with the zoning board. I personally don't want 12 people living across the street from me whether they are too tall, or too short, or on the same basketball team. I think we often create our own difficulties. My experience indicates that the public objects to the density of "handicapped" people imposed by non-integrated service systems, not to "handicapped" people per se.

## REFERENCES

1. *Way To Go.* 1978. University Park Press, Baltimore.

# SOMERSET
# HOME SCHOOL

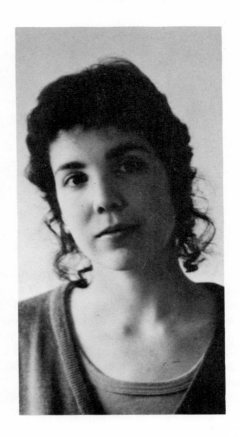

Joanna Cappuccilli

*A child, no matter how disabled, is first and foremost a child.* Although a disability may cause certain differences, he or she is still more like other children than not. All children have characteristics that make them unique, and disabled children are no different. A disability may be one of the characteristics that causes a child to possess an identity separate from those of other children, but being an individual, no matter what your composite, is the way of life.

For children who have more than one disability, life functions may require a great deal of support. But because a child needs assistance is no reason he or she cannot live in a home environment like other children. The home environment may need to be modified and prosthetic equipment may be required, but physically it is possible.

New parents of profoundly disabled children are still often counseled that their child will be a vegetable throughout life. Par-

---

Somerset Home School, 7030 Grant Avenue, Carmichael, CA 95608.

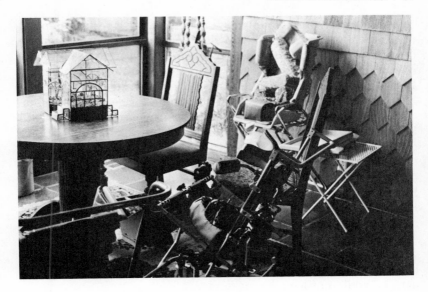

**Figure 1.** There is room for everyone's needs in this dining room.

ents are sometimes told that their disabled child will never learn, never acquire skills, and, essentially, will never grow in any way. Fortunately, however, parents are increasingly beginning to reject this pessimistic perspective. More and more they are realizing that children with disabilities do grow and develop. The steps in their development may be small and their accomplishments may not be giant, but progress can be made and this progress is worth as much as that of a child who plays baseball or who dances ballet.

Perhaps the single most important factor in a child's development is his or her environment. As long as a child lives in a home with love, and is given the proper assistance to learn, the child, no matter how disabled, will grow.

Two years ago, Sarah was in a desperate state. At 18 months she vomited continuously. She had been in the hospital for 30 days and her prognosis looked bleak. She was born with a cyst on her brain and was considered "brain damaged." Her muscles were completely lax. Presumably because of her unusual appearance and her apparently severe mental retardation, doctors felt that recovery was hopeless. The cause of her vomiting was unknown. Her parents were informed that her death was imminent.

A few years ago, John was 2 years old. As a result of spinal meningitis his entire body was rigid. He had numerous seizures daily, suffered from asthma, and screamed incessantly. Unaware of modern treatments for spasticity, his parents kept him on his back. As a result, he developed a severe neck reflex that immobilized his arms. He constantly bit the insides of his cheeks and he was hypersensitive to visitors, mistrusting everyone. His parents felt they had to give him up because they didn't know how to care for him at home.

At 30 months Angie sported an ugly butch haircut as a result of thrashing and rubbing her head. Not only had she worn off her hair, but she had also developed a severe rash over one side of her face. She was blind and extremely emotional. One moment she might be euphoric and the next, hysterical. She did not sleep for more than 2 hours a day, and her body was spastic with severe curvature. When she was angry, which was frequently, she would bite, snarl, and scream. Her mother was not skilled at caring for her and could not keep her at home.

David was profoundly spastic 2 years ago. At 18 months his torso was so severely twisted that his legs were parallel with his neck. He also appeared to be severely mentally retarded. His mother, a single parent with no other children, worked full time. She did not know how to care for David at home, give him the proper attention, and maintain her employment.

Blind and deaf, with a severe muscular disorder and apparent mental retardation, Mark thrashed throughout the night. He never slept, smiled, or cried. He didn't seem to feel pain. At 12 months, he ate only pureed foods and would remain still with his eyes wide open for hours on end. His parents did not feel equipped to help him.

Tommy's disability stemmed from spinal meningitis, undiagnosed for 31 days after a premature birth. He nearly died four times before he left the hospital. At 5 months, when Tommy began to receive physical therapy, he had contractures in his elbows, could not suck, was blind, kept his hands fisted and tucked under his chin, and had no head control.

Tommy's parents were counseled to institutionalize him. They visited the places that had been recommended for their son and could not imagine leaving him in any one of them. Children with disabilities similar to Tommy's were given basic custodial care and left alone for hours without therapy or love and atten-

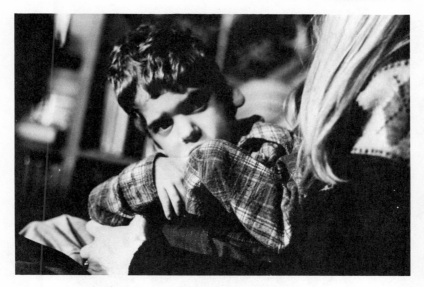

**Figure 2.** Tommy lives at home with his parents.

tion—not because the attendants didn't care, but because there were too many children in one area. They could not find a place where Tommy would receive better care than in their own home. They hoped that Tommy could learn and grow despite his disability, and decided to keep him at home with his older sisters where they could monitor his development and share family love.

Tommy's parents introduced prosthetic devices and training programs to counteract the effects of his disability and to give him opportunities to strive for the small successes his abilities permitted. He received physical therapy, which included positioning and feeding techniques. Because little was known about the treatment of children like Tommy, his parents spent many hours searching for appropriate program methods. They made some mistakes, but they also made many discoveries.

Unfortunately, it is unusual for children with Tommy's level of disability to be given this opportunity. Children with similar disabilities often go untreated. They are allowed to remain for days in one position and as a result develop open sores, deformities, and contractures. At 6 years of age, Tommy's original contractures are gone, he can use his hands, he has some head control, and he visually tracks objects—not bad for a child who once had

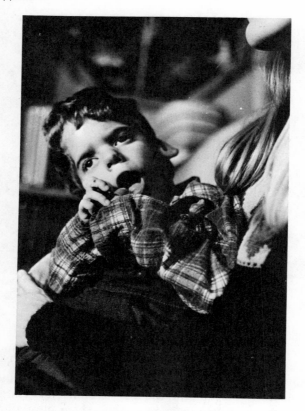

**Figure 3.** Tommy is eating table foods and using his hands.

no vision! Tommy is eating table foods and is almost toilet trained. His warm personality is very unique; he shows love and affection. His sisters, Lisa and Jill, are very proud of him.

Tommy's parents, Tom Senior and Sunny Whalley, became aware of other youngsters with similar disabilities while trying to find appropriate assistance and treatment for Tommy. Their awareness and interest expanded, and in 1976 they opened Somerset Home School, a concept in living and learning for young children up to 6 years old who have multiple disabilities.

Conceived as a community-based home for children who could not be placed elsewhere, the Whalleys give severely disabled children a chance to develop their full potential. Somerset Home School operates to help children function to the best of their abil-

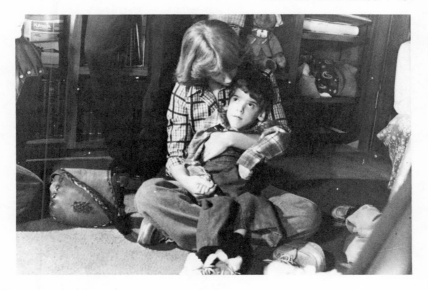

**Figure 4.** His sister Lisa is proud of Tommy.

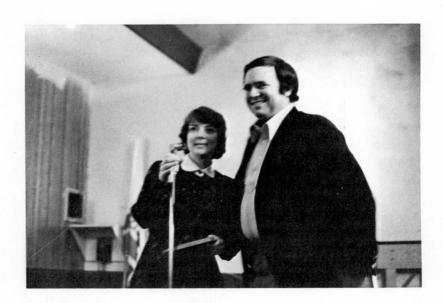

**Figure 5.** Tom and Sunny Whalley, founders of Somerset.

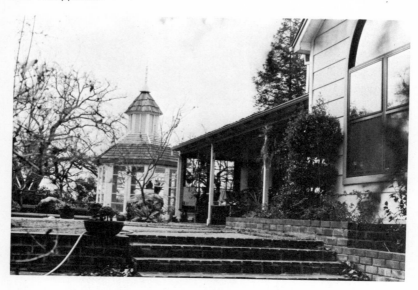

**Figure 6.** Somerset, a scenic environment.

ity, even if this means merely eating without vomiting or sleeping soundly through the night.

Programming for the children takes place around the clock and is based on the concept that children with severe disabilities can be taught more than is traditionally expected. Daily activities are enriching and provide the kinds of experiences that an average preschooler gets. They include such events as swimming in a specially built pool, riding on the family pony, and listening to music. In addition, the children are taught skills that lead to self-dependence, such as biting, chewing, muscle movements, and toilet training. The Somerset Home atmosphere allows the children to develop their senses through natural stimulation, i.e., family interaction, bathroom and kitchen smells, and touching various textures.

The Somerset environment is picturesque and comfortable. The children live in the Whalley family home near Sacramento, California. The rooms are decorative and warm, and the children are treated as part of the family, living and dining in the Whalley's spacious kitchen and living room. Outside, the children find a variety of colors, noises, and surfaces, including the greenness of grass, the sounds of birds, and the tickle of a ladybug on their hands.

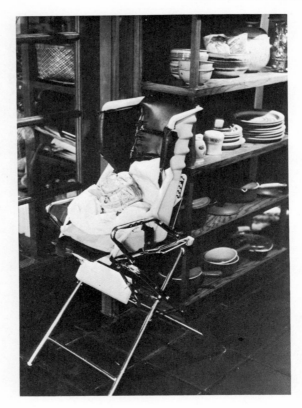

**Figure 7.** Specially modified chairs for dining help make Somerset a comfortable place to live.

An important component of Somerset is that parents continue to be involved with their children. They are encouraged to visit their children weekly and to take them home for vacations. The parents are trained to care for their children in the same way as the staff is. It is hoped that most of the children will eventually be able to return to their natural homes.

Sarah, John, Angie, David, and Mark have all lived at Somerset for approximately 2 years. Each benefits tremendously from this experience. Their progress and growth is subtle and often slow relative to other standards, but their success is a testimony to the Whalleys' faith in their progress.

Today, Sarah is 3½ years old. She has progressed incredibly. It was learned that her vomiting was due to a food allergy. With

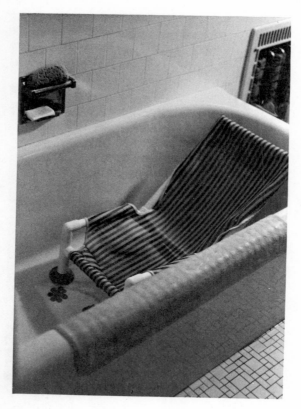

**Figure 8.**   Any bathroom will do.

proper diet, Sarah's problem is now under control. Initially near death, she has transformed into a babbling little girl with personality and sparkle. Massaged daily and kept very warm, Sarah's muscles are still lax but she is beginning to use her hands. Progress has been rapid for this pretty blonde girl.

Sun soothes John and his traumatic episodes have vanished. With red lights and Tschaikowsky, John has learned to sleep through the night, to laugh, show contentment, and to hum in perfect pitch! John is beginning to obtain head control and develop some vision. His asthma is now controlled and his seizure frequency is considerably reduced. A regular routine, proper medication, and minimal emotional stress at Somerset have encouraged a beautiful boy to appear from behind the frightened child who ex-

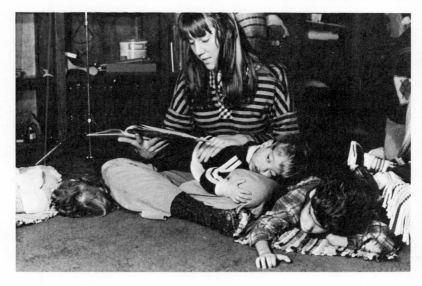

**Figure 9.** Sensory development is an important component of Somerset programming.

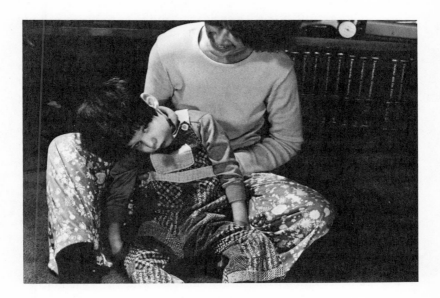

**Figure 10.** John is beginning to learn head control.

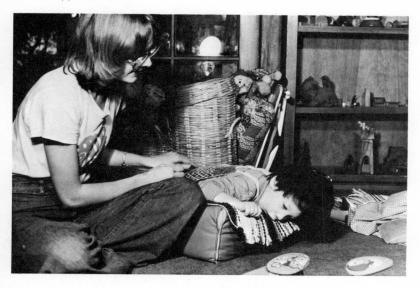

**Figure 11.** John's traumatic episodes have vanished.

isted 2 years ago. Now 4 years old, John stands with support and observes life around him with curiosity, giving as well as receiving love.

Angie, at 4½, still has periods of anger, but only when anger is appropriate. The Whalleys know Angie so well that they can often predict and prevent her anger. Today Angie is soothed by music and sunshine and has come a very long way toward being like other children.

David's mother has learned enough to care for him at home every weekend. She is elated by his progress. David understands a great deal and hears and sees everything around him. His unique personality makes him a joy to be around.

Now 3 years old, Mark has also made remarkable progress. He has learned to smile and cry appropriately, his seizures have decreased considerably, and he sleeps well. He has learned to swim, and even to walk. Still unable to speak, he has spontaneously developed sign language. Although still hard of hearing, he is the most mobile of all the children at Somerset. Fun to be with, Mark is a comedian and an individual who adds his own share of love to the Whalley family life.

All of these children were considered medically fragile when they first moved to Somerset. Now they have outgrown this cate-

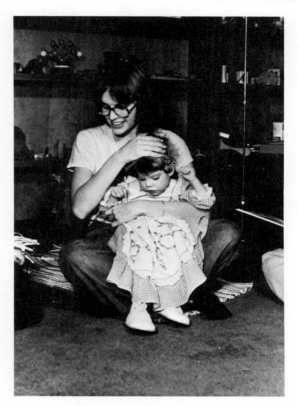

**Figure 12.** Angie's anger can be predicted and prevented.

gory. They share sibling affection (when one cries, the others, apparently in sympathy, cry too) and they seem to communicate with one another without words. Routine, love, and systematic therapy are Somerset's keys to success.

Somerset is a challenge and a creative project. Its directors are pioneers. Reward for their efforts comes to the Whalleys in actualizing the positive predictions they have made for the potential of their children. Unfortunately, Somerset does not receive the level of support the state offers to large institutional facilities.

After surviving a discouraging application process for licensure, Somerset finally received a state license. A private facility could have easily been opened to serve children from wealthy families, but the directors were steadfast in making Somerset available to all children. After many challenging ordeals, and with

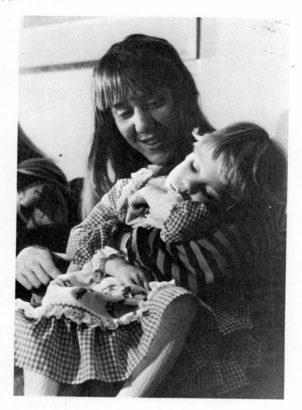

**Figure 13.** Music and sunshine soothe Angie.

great persistence, a special monthly rate was secured through the Regional Center System. Meanwhile, state institutions are operated at a much higher rate. The Whalleys are able to pay their staff only because they do not pay themselves. Payments on the home, food, and other expenses must come from Tom's full-time engineering work. The state will temporarily offer increased amounts for children placed in their home directly from state hospitals, but less support is provided for children who need temporary out-of-home placements.

Originally, it was hoped that most of the children would return to their natural families. The directors now realize that although some children will go home, others will not. The currently

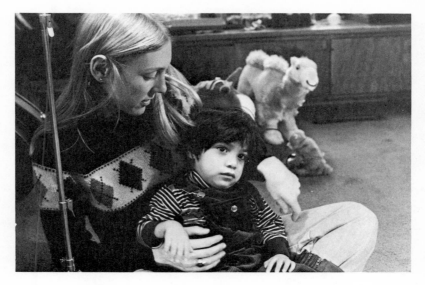

**Figure 14.** David hears and sees everything around him.

available placement options for these children are difficult to accept. Few alternatives, other than placement in an institution for the severely disabled, are to be found. The Whalleys are convinced that, without continued programming, the children will regress and develop many of the anomalies of older children and adults who have similar disabilities.

Sunny and Tom encourage others to open homes like theirs. They also encourage foster and adoptive parents who are willing to raise children like Angie, Sarah, and Mark. More important, they hope support services will be available to natural parents so that they may never have to send their children away for treatment. The Whalleys have directly contributed to generating alternative settings by recently opening a new home for 6- to 12-year-old children with severe disabilities. This new home will accept children like Libby, 9, who has been staying at Somerset for a few months while waiting to move into a new program. Libby previously lived in another group home where the staff was not sensitive to her needs. Although previously toilet trained, Libby was made to wear diapers. She was force-fed pureed foods through a tube and was not put into an educational program because the

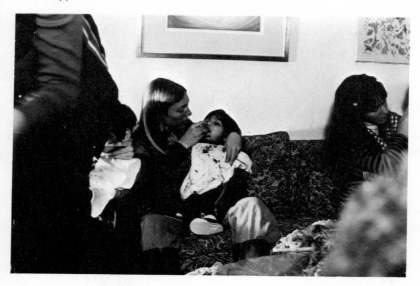

**Figure 15.** Enjoying a piece of chocolate cake at Christmas.

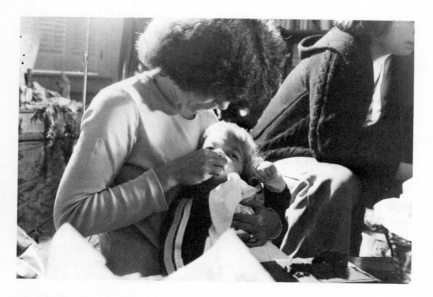

**Figure 16.** Mark loves eating.

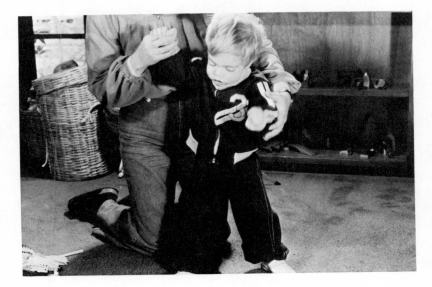

**Figure 17.** Mark swims and walks, the most mobile of the children at Somerset.

staff was unaware that she could learn. She frequently had hysterical outbreaks.

It has been found that Libby has no need for diapers and enjoys eating mashed table foods. She can tell time and read, skills which she apparently learned on her own. She has never had an emotional outburst during her 7-month stay at Somerset. Those who have been to Somerset are convinced that Libby's growth is due to having lived in a normal home, where she is respected for what she can do and assisted when necessary.

The Somerset waiting list grows longer each month. Current laws mandate all of the services provided at Somerset. The widespread application of these legal regulations, however, is taking a great deal of time. Thus, the Whalleys face an uphill climb toward establishing a normal life for themselves and the children they serve. While the Whalleys enjoy their work and look forward to a continued effort in the years ahead, they hope to see the day when more options are available for children like Tommy.

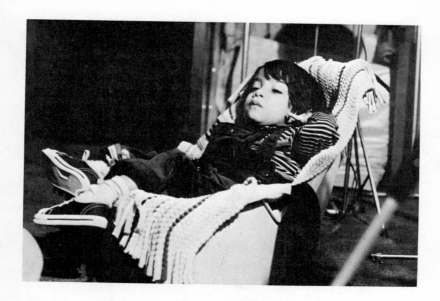

**Figure 19.** It is hoped that more homes like Somerset will be developed for other children with needs like David's.

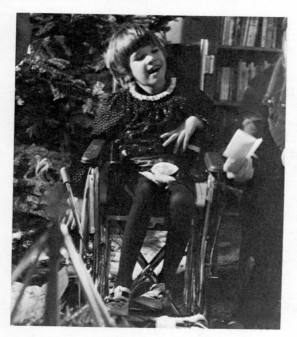

**Figure 18.** Libby, on the road to learning self-help.

# PERSONAL ADVOCACY

## A Model to Equalize Consumer Power

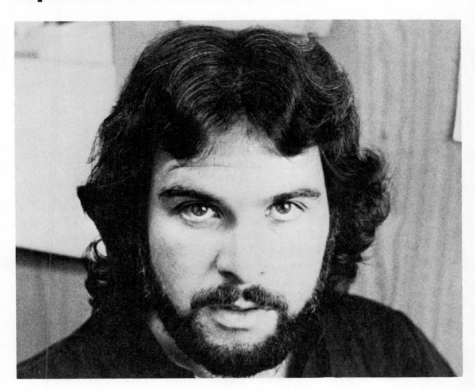

Albert Zonca

*In* *recent* *years,* *there* *has* *been* *a* *growing*
awareness of and appreciation for the human and civil rights of
persons with developmental disabilities. Services that assist developmentally disabled citizens in minimizing their disabilities
and maximizing their potential have increasingly been regarded
as a legitimate right rather than a privilege. Class advocacy efforts have netted significant results in the areas of legislation and
litigation, granting developmentally disabled persons the legal
rights to education, habilitation, and the opportunity to live as
first class citizens with all the attendant rights and benefits. This
has lent impetus to the deinstitutionalization of many persons
with developmental handicaps, and their subsequent return to our
communities, where, theoretically, they will have the opportunity
to live more normal, meaningful lives participating in the mainstream culture.

Because class advocacy efforts have brought about major
changes in the last 25 years, in many ways we have attached
greater significance and importance to systems and class advo-

cacy (advocacy on behalf of developmentally disabled persons as a population group) than to individual personal advocacy. Systems change is needed—it is both necessary and beneficial. Class action can often have a greater impact than individual action. However, we have failed much of the time to assist *individuals* with developmental disabilities in actualizing the accomplishments and great gains we have made at the class level. In our preoccupation with the needs of persons with developmental disabilities as a group, we have neglected to develop mechanisms to assist the *individual* developmentally disabled consumer acquire what he or she may personally need to improve the quality of his or her life.

This reality should be obvious to everyone directly involved with primary consumers. The great court decisions of the past 10 years have not yet had much impact on many disabled citizens, nor has the rhetoric of new federal and state laws been transformed into tangible reality. Despite the great advances we are so proud of, many developmentally disabled persons still are not receiving a "free and appropriate education," nor living in the "least restrictive alternative," nor obtaining the "habilitation" they need. I could give countless examples of developmentally disabled persons whose rights have been abridged to varying degrees— sometimes by the institutions in which they live, or by the agencies designed to serve them, or sometimes, sadly, by members of their own families.

There are a variety of factors that inhibit persons with developmental disabilities from actualizing their legal and human rights. Of primary importance, of course, is the disability itself and the vulnerability it often creates in the individual. Persons with intellectual impairment have greater difficulty understanding and navigating in a society so incredibly complex and requiring increasing intellectual expertise and sophistication in so many areas. Persons with impaired intellectual capacity are at a distinct, obvious disadvantage in functioning successfully in such a culture. Other handicapping conditions, cerebral palsy, for example, may hamper effective speech or physical dexterity. For many persons, the deficits of intellectual impairment are exacerbated by accompanying physical handicaps. A further complicating factor occurs for people who, because of long-term institutionalization, have been isolated physically and socially from society. Their ability to function within society is then further impaired by their separation from the mainstream culture. This process of institutionalization, along with society's accompanying attitudes about persons who have disabilities, has served to condition developmentally disabled individuals to helplessness. Many developmentally disabled persons have low self-esteem and fail to recognize their own individuality and worth. They have not been given the message that it is "okay" to have needs and to express those needs. They, perhaps more than any other individual group, have been taught to be non-assertive and nondemanding. The combined result of all of these factors is a degree of dependency that is antithetical to self-representation and effective advocacy. The developmentally disabled person is left more vulnerable and is less likely to be in a position to represent his or her interests effectively.

In recent years, there has been a tremendous growth in human services in an attempt to implement various laws designed to include previously disenfranchised citizens. Bureaucracy has grown uncontrollably in size and into an extremely impersonal system of outmoded rules and organizational rigidity. The human services bureaucracy has been repeatedly criticized for its unresponsiveness and lack of accountability to clients. In the developmental disabilities field, we have seen the proliferation of organizations at all geographical levels—national, multi-state, state, regional, and local. Ron Neufeld, in his paper "Advocacy and the Human Service Delivery System" (1), captures well what this "system" must seem like to the consumer. He compares the service system to a giant maze:

> The maze runners are not rats, but humans who are trying to obtain the services and resources which are the reinforcers at the end of the maze. One gets the feeling that only a very small proportion of the total reinforcers or resources set aside for disabled persons are dispersed to them. The largest proportion of the resources are absorbed in maintaining organizations that exist in and for themselves. In keeping with Darwinian theory, only the fittest maze runners survive. In this system, handicapped people are always the losers. Maybe that is what advocacy is all about—trying to minimize the losses for developmentally disabled citizens.

A variety of service delivery agencies have been created that are designated to provide support to developmentally disabled consumers and to assist them in navigating this maze. However, these agencies too have been subject to bureaucratization, or what more astutely has been called "bureaupathology." Agencies that were created to perform collective social work functions, have, because of bureaucratization, become grossly perverted from their original intent. It is ironic that today so many social workers are attempting to rediscover advocacy. The pioneers in the social work movement clearly defined their role as one of change agent and advocate. Their very reason for existence was to ensure that more vulnerable individuals in society had the opportunity for a better life. The development of formalized, rigid structures have today relegated many social workers to being bureaucratic "gate keepers," ensuring that only the "right" people with the "right" problems are served. Accountability requirements, although well intentioned, have consumed increasing amounts of time and generated seemingly endless paperwork. This means staff time is *removed* from the individual consumer and is spent justifying service plans, rather than helping the individual obtain what he or she needs.

Conflict of interest issues also have been well outlined in the past 10 years and there is at least an increased consciousness and clearer conceptualization of the problem. A variety of factors bind those within human service agencies and diminish their freedom to be advocates for their clients. For example, internal pressures, agency policies, and the demands of other clients can all inhibit effective advocacy at this level.

## SONOMA COUNTY ADVOCACY SYSTEM

Why in a book of this nature, dedicated primarily to presenting various residential models, is it appropriate to address the issue of advocacy and advocacy systems? Any system, residential or otherwise, regardless of how benevolent or well intentioned, will be subject to certain basic human and organizational dilemmas that have an adverse effect on its ability to keep the client's interests primary. In planning and implementing any system of service, it is paramount that we simultaneously address the issues of protecting those individuals to be served.

For the past year, in Sonoma County, California, we have been implementing a multidimensional personal advocacy system to attempt to provide that protective safeguard. It is but one model, whose deficits and strengths will more clearly emerge over time. It incorporates the strengths of a variety of protection and advocacy schemata that have been successful.

Advocacy mechanisms can be of basically two kinds, external or internal. Internal advocacy originates in, is supported by, and operates from within some service system. External advocacy is independent of such a system and works outside it. There are, of course, strengths and weaknesses in both approaches and divergent points of view about the relative merits of each. An internal advocate is paid by the system in which she or he works and is committed in some way to identifying persons within that system whose rights and needs are not being met. Internal advocates try to negotiate within the system to bring about effective change that will assist the client. This valuable and needed approach can be quite effective in resolving individual problems for consumers. However, internal advocates are only free to act with the sanction of the system in which they operate. Internal advocates are faced with a serious threat of co-option, because their social contacts, their professional identity, their salary, etc., are all tied to the agency they serve. They are always at risk of internalizing the agency "point of view" in a conflict with a client rather than the client "point of view." Systems tend to resist change, and when they have control over the change agent, they often actualize that resistance by weakening the agent's ability to act. Because of this resistance, there are those who claim that internal advocacy is indeed not advocacy at all—that changes occur only because of the *outside* forces impacting on the agency or system.

The Sonoma County Personal Advocacy System utilizes an external advocacy approach. It receives no financial support from sources with which it may find itself in an advocacy arena. It is organized as a nonprofit corporation with a broadly based board of directors representing the community and various disability interests. There are seven sources of funding, all remote from local and state service providers. Over half of the budget is supported by federal funds received or administered either through the California Protection and Advocacy System or the Regional Developmental Disability Office of HEW. These funds are specifically provided to encourage and support advocacy activity for developmentally disabled persons. The realities of organizational dynamics dictate that *external* forces are often needed to move complex bureaucratic organizations and systems. Because of his or her autonomy, the external advocate is less likely to be co-opted or stopped. The external advocate has greater freedom to push as hard, as long, and as often as necessary to create the desired result. There are, of course, disadvantages to this approach. External advocates are most often still viewed as adversaries, rather than necessary catalysts to change. This creates a lack of trust and makes it difficult for external advocates to get necessary information. It also is much more difficult for external advocacy organizations to find funding because most funding sources are in some way tied to the service delivery system. Even those that at first glance do not appear to be directly tied to the system often are in some way and can dilute advocacy in more subtle ways. Accountability and other requirements, for example, can bureaucratize external advocacy organization to such a degree that it loses much of its autonomy and freedom to act.

Sonoma County has more than 10,000 people with developmental disabilities. Approximately 1,800 of these individuals reside at Sonoma State Hospital, a massive 80-building facility located in a rural area of the county. The remaining individuals with developmental handicaps are living in various areas of the county: some with families, others in residential care facilities or group homes, and still others in more independent settings. Classically, persons with developmental disabilities in Sonoma County, as elsewhere, continue to receive neither the quantity nor the quality of service they need to become truly participating members of society. Their social condition is a microcosm of the problems persons with developmental handicaps encounter throughout the country.

## Citizen Advocacy

In 1973, Sonoma County Citizen Advocacy, Inc., began operation of a Citizen Advocacy program whereby volunteers are matched on a one-to-one basis with persons with developmental disabilities. Citizen volunteers are recruited, screened, trained, and monitored to serve as personal advocates for developmentally disabled individuals who need assistance in ensuring that their rights and interests are protected. This concept was developed in Nebraska in 1970 and has now spread throughout the nation and Canada.

Advocates fill a variety of roles and functions, such as serving as liaisons with government and/or private agencies on behalf of developmentally disabled persons; assisting in solving problems regarding transportation, housing and shopping; helping with property and income management; representing consumer interests vis-à-vis agencies and the law; ensuring receipt of other appropriate services; and becoming payees, guardians, or conservators. Citizen advocates also assist developmentally disabled persons in learning techniques that will enable them to become more adept in the future in advocating for themselves. The advocate assists the developmentally disabled person in defending his or her rights and interests while providing practical guidance as well as the emotional support so often missing in the highly impersonal bureaucratic protection and service delivery mechanisms.

After 4 years of operation, the program, although highly successful, was unable to meet the demand for personal advocates requested. It became apparent that, regardless of how efficient program operation was and how many staff members were added, there was a variety of external factors limiting the number of personal advocates available at any one time in our community. Sonoma County has a population of roughly 300,000 people living in a mixture of rural, suburban, and small city settings. The county has a large number of local human service agencies and organizations that utilize volunteers in their programs. They have inundated the population with requests for volunteer assistance. This is a highly positive phenomenon from the volunteer's perspective, in that the volunteer has more options. However, from the perspective of a citizen advocacy program, it makes recruitment all the more difficult and limits the number of people available at any given time.

In addition, a variety of socio-cultural factors have had a profound impact on volunteerism as of late. The increased number of working women, for example, has diminished their availability as a volunteer resource pool. In addition, not all people who need advocacy intervention need full-time citizen advocates. Some could better use short-term intervention; others can effectively represent their rights and interests, given the confidence and training. The citizen advocacy model was never intended to be *the* solution to all needs at the personal advocacy level. In the Sonoma County Personal Advocacy System, citizen advocacy is utilized as one component of a multidimensional advocacy continuum.

The Sonoma County Personal Advocacy System builds on the citizen advocacy schema and includes the additional components of self-advocacy, affiliative (parental) advocacy, and broker advocacy.

## The Self-Advocacy Component

The Accreditation Council for Facilities for the Mentally Retarded states that self-advocacy is the "presentation of the rights and interests of one's self to bring about change, in order that barriers in meeting identified needs be overcome . . . all developmentally disabled persons should be provided an opportunity to reach the most desirable level of advocacy which is self-preservation, an inherent right'' (1).

Persons with developmental disabilities often lack the skills and awareness necessary for self-advocating behavior, and frequently respond to the expectations of others who assume that a developmentally disabled person's intellectual limitations prevent him from understanding or even knowing his needs and feelings, much less being able to assert himself. As a result, many handicapped persons learn to respond to pressure and coercion with submissive and acquiescent behavior.

We have designed self-advocacy training to teach consumers appropriate assertive responses and afford them the opportunity to practice these responses in a supportive environment. The training is based on the assumption that, if non-assertive behavior can be learned, it can also be unlearned and replaced with newly acquired behavior. Many individuals with developmental disabilities can, with proper support, learn to better represent their rights and interests. This has not occurred because it is an area of instruction that has been sorely neglected. For example, there is little information on rights, services, or developmental disability planning that is disseminated in other than a fairly sophisticated and complex format. As a result, the very information that most significantly affects the developmentally disabled consumer is not accessible to the consumer in a form that he or she can readily understand and utilize. Developmentally disabled persons can, with proper assistance, learn about their legal rights and the developmental disabilities mega-system, and how to assume more control over their own lives.

We are currently testing two training modules of eight sessions each. They utilize a format of group discussion, didactic presentations, various behavior rehearsal techniques, such as modeling and role playing, and structured practice exercises. Video- and audiotaping is used to give immediate feedback on behavior in simulated situations, enabling participants to monitor their strengths and weaknesses in self-advocacy roles, and to modify their behavior accordingly. Material designed particularly for consumers with developmental disabilities is being developed. Some materials are taped, others written in simple language, and still others are illustrated.

Groups are composed of six to eight persons, an optimum setting for participants to practice and internalize the concepts presented. The targets for this component are adults who are verbal and mildly or moderately disabled.

## The Parent Advocacy Component

Young children cannot advocate for themselves. Parents are the legitimate advocates for their children. Their advocacy is highly effective because the affiliative relationship creates strong natural and personal bonds and motivations. Parents of handicapped children have traditionally been viewed as their children's advocates, often even after their offspring have reached adulthood. Parents have collectively organized voluntary associations and other advocacy groups that have been catalysts for change in the disability rights movement.

Some parents, through years of learning and struggling, have become highly sophisticated and knowledgeable advocates. However, this expertise often takes years to develop. The parents of a newly identified disabled child are suddenly catapulted into an area totally unfamiliar and often overwhelming. Sometimes, years of adjustment and learning pass before the parents become truly effective advocates for the child. Sometimes this never occurs. It is critical that children receive the services they need as early as possible, in order to maximize their potential for optimal growth and development. The sooner the parent can become an effective advocate for his or her child, the greater will be the impact on that child's life.

Parent advocacy training can maximize the parent's effectiveness as an advocate. Just as primary consumers with developmental disabilities often do not have access to information about rights and services designed especially for them, so too are parents frequently without this vital information. Much material available within the existing network of information sharing is designed for and channeled to professionals and those few parents who are well entrenched in the developmental disabilities system. Information can and should be shared with *all* parents of developmentally disabled children.

Parents can also be taught techniques and strategies that will enable them to better acquire services and effectively mobilize the system to meet the needs of their children. Many parents are intimidated by professionals and by an arena with unfamiliar language and a highly complex structure. They must be taught to know the system and its jargon, to know their own and their children's rights within that system, and to exercise their rights as natural advocates for their children.

Training utilizes a variety of teaching techniques, including group discussions, lectures, tapes, slides, films, and demonstrations. Training includes information regarding the service delivery system, developmental disabilities legislation, relevant litigation, research techniques, advocacy techniques and strategies, normalization, and information about the various handicapping conditions. An extensive library is available for parents to do their own research after they have been trained.

Parents who have completed the training, have internalized the concepts and skills presented, and have demonstrated an exemplary adjustment to their handicapped children are selected to become members of a parent advocacy council. The parent advocacy council serves as a mechanism whereby trained parents are available to other parents to provide support, furnish information regarding the parent movement and professional services and programs, and mobilize groups of parents on specific advocacy issues on behalf of their handicapped children.

## The Broker Advocacy Component

Not all handicapped persons have involved parents who can effectively advocate for them. Occasionally, parents reach impasses where they cannot continue alone without the help of someone with greater expertise. Moreover, individuals with developmental disabilities, even those who can learn to effectively advocate for themselves, still may need to rely on a representative to intervene in times of crisis and particular confusion. Others with more severe handicaps may rely on such a representative more frequently. Citizen advocates can fill this role, but they also at times need to rely on a more knowledgeable person for assistance.

California state hospitals and regional centers for the developmentally disabled have provided client's rights representatives to assist individuals within those systems. However, such in-house advocates are controlled by the service system and are only free to effectively advocate for developmentally disabled individuals to the extent the system permits. The Sonoma County Personal Advocacy System utilizes a personal representative who, at the request of the developmentally disabled person and/or his or her family, can serve as an agent to negotiate for needed services. The broker is paralegally trained and competent to negotiate and bargain on behalf of the developmentally disabled persons. The process of negotiating for services in the marketplace is a promising coordination technique. A broker can produce unique combinations of services that are not available through regular serving systems. In a sense, the broker can be a catalyst for effective service delivery.

This objective is clearly related to a series of recommendations the President's Committee on Mental Retardation made in its major report, "Mental Retardation; Century of Decision; A Report to the President" (2). These recommendations propose that every mentally retarded person who wishes or requires one will be assured the opportunity and means to select or employ an agency or agent as a personal representative to negotiate on his or her behalf for any available service required, no matter how brief or extended the service may be.

Assistance is provided by the broker on either a sustained or episodic basis, depending on the nature and the need for assistance. The broker's role is clearly delineated as a representative function, that is, one of helping to secure services and related benefits and not one of supplying those benefits directly. Services include information and referral, counseling, representation and intervention, and paralegal assistance. There are currently five volunteer attorneys who are available to assist the broker with legal questions and issues and assist developmentally disabled consumers with low or no cost legal aid when necessary.

In the event that the broker is not able to achieve the necessary outcome for the consumer, he or she works with the existing service delivery system to try to overcome whatever barrier or problem is preventing the consumer from receiving what he or she needs. The broker observes and documents gaps in services, or service rigidity, which inhibit response to the needs of individuals, and then works with other agencies to help resolve systemic problems.

## CONCLUSION

In its first year of operation, the Sonoma County Personal Advocacy System provided services to more than 800 developmentally disabled persons and/or their families. The use of its services by primary and secondary consumers has been overwhelming. Requests were primarily for assistance in dealing with agencies designed to serve developmentally disabled persons who, from the consumers' perspective, were derelict in that function. The four components of citizen advocacy, self-advocacy, parent advocacy, and broker advocacy have allowed maximum flexibility in responding to individual consumer requests.

There has been, of course, resistance from human service professionals who claim they are already "doing advocacy" and that our service is a duplication. Some political bodies in the beginning resisted cooperation on grounds of legitimacy. We have had to demonstrate that "legitimacy" does not come only from government sanction.

Despite this resistance, however, the advantages of such an approach are becoming clearly evident. In a time of disenchantment with bureaucratic sprawl, the merits of smaller, more responsive organizations are being viewed with more seriousness. Individuals who are being served identify strongly with such organizations because they receive more efficient and effective assistance than they do from large bureaucratic organizations. They do not identify with the bureaucracy because that is usually where they encounter the greatest difficulty, and certainly the greatest depersonalization.

We are at a new stage in the development of organizations and systems to implement social policy. As a society, we have become more aware of the deficits of bureaucracy. Our elevated consciousness is reflected in recent legislation, which addresses the need for protective mechanisms that will ensure bureaucracy does what it was designed to do—*serve people*. As a result, all over the country we are beginning to grope for new social mechanisms. The Sonoma County Personal Advocacy System is one approach. It is not important that this model be implemented throughout the country. What is important is that in designing service systems in the future we become sensitized to the need to include in our designs appropriate advocacy mechanisms that are free of conflict of interest and accessible both geographically and economically to developmentally disabled consumers and their families. As these organizations become increasingly successful in serving consumers, public consciousness of their usefulness will be elevated and consumers will increasingly mobilize to ensure their continuance. Advocacy mechanisms will then be perceived as legitimate and necessary means to equalize the power of the consumer and diminish his or her vulnerability when dealing with bureaucracy.

## REFERENCES

1. Neufeld, G. R. 1977. Advocacy and the human service delivery system. Developmental Disability Technical Assistance System, Chapel Hill, N.C.
2. President's Committee on Mental Retardation. 1976. Mental Retardation; Century of Decision; A Report to the President. U.S. Government Printing Office, Washington, D.C.

# THE
# PENNSYLVANIA
# SYSTEM

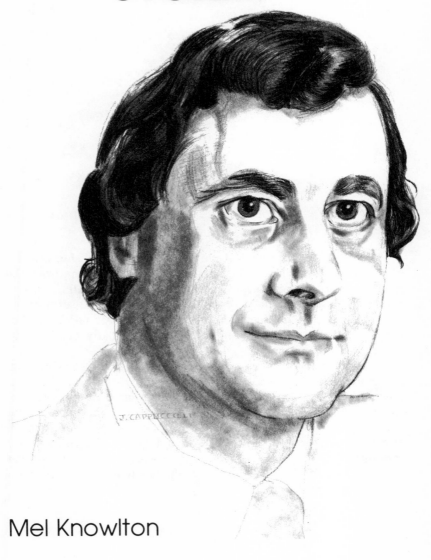

## Mel Knowlton

*The community service system that we are creating* in Pennsylvania is not dramatically different from the models described for Macomb-Oakland and ENCOR. All three systems represent attempts to create normalizing social services for persons with special needs. Pennsylvania's client needs and its program models are very similar to those already outlined for Michigan and Nebraska.

I agree wholeheartedly with the overall service design concepts presented by Gerald Provencal and Wade Hitzing. In order not to be repetitive, I focus in this chapter on related considerations drawn from our experience in Pennsylvania, specifically: 1) the background of Pennsylvania's Community Service System, 2) the system's components, 3) Pennsylvania's efforts to create community-based, alternative living concepts for citizens with special needs, and 4) two major problems currently facing Pennsylvania's service system.

## BACKGROUND

A massive movement was begun in 1972 by the Pennsylvania Association for Retarded Citizens to create less restrictive environments for Pennsylvania's mentally retarded citizens. The first funding breakthrough occurred in April, 1972, when the Pennsylvania Office of Mental Retardation received $1.9 million from the Pennsylvania General Assembly. We then had about 12,500 people living in institutions. Pennsylvania's public institutions now house approximately 8,000 clients. We have pushed to move institutionalized children back to their natural homes and to help institutionalized adults live independently. We have had 2,000 people move into one of these two options over the past 5½ years and we are proud of this record.

We stress two factors in addressing the needs of our client population: deinstitutionalization and the prevention of institutionalization. We have maintained a policy for the past 4 years that 50% of all new community placements must come from an institution, with the remaining 50% from the community. We modified our policy this year so that now 80% must come from institutions and 20% from the community. We do have a waiver clause, however. If a particular county goes over its 20% allotment it does not have to send someone from the community into an institution for a week so that the person may receive a community space. Our percentage quotas are guidelines that we strongly encourage counties to follow. Exceptions are permitted.

Our primary residential priority in Pennsylvania is to identify and deliver services that permit clients to live at home. We support respite services, family training and education, homemaker services, in-home support services, transportation, leisure time activities, and recreational experiences. As a second priority we provide adoptive and foster home services. These settings receive the same ancillary services delivered to natural families. Our emphasis is on providing small, highly integrated living arrangements.

## SYSTEMIC ORGANIZATION AND SERVICE DESIGN

### Organization

Pennsylvania has an Office of Mental Retardation within its Department of Public Welfare. There are three bureaus under the

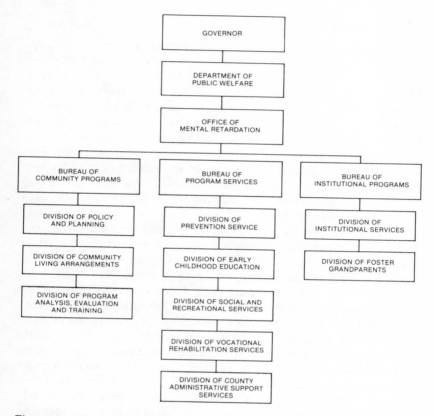

**Figure 1.** Organization of Pennsylvania's Office of Mental Retardation.

Office of Mental Retardation: 1) the Bureau of Community Programs, 2) the Bureau of Program Services, and 3) the Bureau of Institutional Programs. Community-based residential services are managed through the Bureau of Community Programs. Figure 1 depicts the overall organizational structure for the Office of Mental Retardation.

The various levels of authority and responsibility for Pennsylvania's mental retardation service delivery are shown in Figure 2. The Office of Mental Retardation is responsible for program standards, policy decisions, budgetary funding approval, evaluation, staff training, and program consultation. Additionally, Pennsylvania is divided into four regional, state-operated offices.

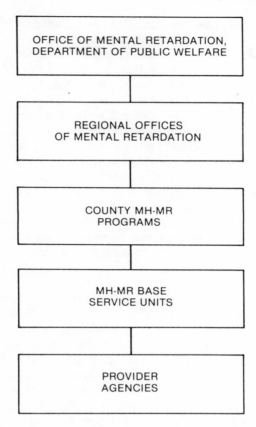

**Figure 2.** Levels of authority/responsibility for Pennsylvania's Service Delivery System.

Regional offices are responsible for program approval, monitoring program quality and outcomes, program evaluation, and staff training. The roles of the state office and its regional offices overlap and appear to necessitate frequent redefinition because of changes in policies and program standards.

The county level of Pennsylvania's complex human services design is responsible for the provision of mental health and mental retardation services. We have 41 mental health/mental retardation units for 67 counties, so some counties have joined together to form one unit. Local catchment areas, called Base Service Units, are charged with overseeing admission releases, active treatment plans, case management, and diagnosis. Base Service Units may directly deliver services or may purchase services, such as community living arrangements, from provider agencies.

Monies are sent from the state to the counties. Most counties opt to contract with not-for-profit proprietors for services. In the area of community living arrangements we have only three providers who operate on profit-based accounting systems and five county units that directly operate programs. I might add that from our experience there is no difference in program cost or quality among not-for-profit, profit, and county-operated programs.

As the titles of its organizational units imply, Pennsylvania's service system is categorically organized. It exists specifically to meet the needs of people who are labeled "mentally retarded." Clients who have secondary problems, such as sensory impairments, cerebral palsy, and emotional problems, may also receive services provided that their primary diagnosis is "mental retardation."

## Service Options

Pennsylvania has developed a continuum of residential services that is flexible and structured to meet the needs of all mentally retarded individuals, no matter what the age or severity of handicap. The following list shows the services offered through Pennsylvania's Office of Mental Retardation. The first category, Family Resource Services, refers to the range of things we do to help natural families maintain their handicapped son or daughter at home. The degree to which these services are implemented is defined by county priorities and depends on the availability of funds.

**Family Resource Services**
    Visiting nurse services
    Family respite
    Family training and education
    Homemaker services
    In-home support
    Transportation
    Leisure time activities/recreation

**Adoptive Home and Foster Home Services**
    Visiting nurse services
    Family respite
    Family training and education

Homemaker services
In-home support
Transportation
Leisure time activities/recreation

If a child cannot stay with his or her natural family, we supply the same level of services to the child and his or her support system in the context of an adoptive or foster home. Some foster parents eventually adopt "mentally retarded" children. Initial foster placement provides the child and foster parents with an opportunity to get acquainted before adoption.

Our Community Living Arrangement (CLA) Program is now in its sixth year. We initially designed this program like the ENCOR model but have since tailored it to meet the specific needs of our situation in Pennsylvania. All CLA staff members work for the service provider under contract with the county or director for the county. No foster parents are involved. All living settings are leased by the service provider.

Our service for individuals who are medically complex and multiply handicapped is known as the Developmental Maximation Unit. Three of these that are currently in operation house between 20 and 30 medically fragile individuals in skilled intermediate nursing home facilities. We are beginning to serve this group of clients in small homes and apartments with either nurses living in or on call to the regular live-in staff.

Another service that we offer, intensive habit shaping, is for children and adults with severe problems in areas like head hitting, eating, and toileting. It is a short-term program of behavioral correction. We attempt to offer these services in an apartment or home with only a single severely handicapped individual present and up to two more clients who are not severely handicapped.

We serve most children from birth through 18 years old in our Child Development Program. The children typically have a wide range of medical and behavioral problems. Three out of four children reside in a house or apartment, with no more than one person demonstrating severe problems. We teach skills learned in normal living settings, such as toothbrushing, washing, and dressing.

The structured correctional program is for individuals who have problems with society. This is generally the juvenile or adult retarded offender who needs a short-term, structured, and intensely supervised residential setting. These settings are usually small homes or apartments where a trained staff works with the retarded client to help facilitate his or her readjustment to society.

Most adults receive one of two interrelated services: adult training, delivered in a small group living arrangement; or adult minimal supervision, delivered in the context of the client's independent living setting. Adult training is offered in group homes or apartments with three or fewer clients. Emphasis is placed on teaching clients independent living skills. Clients may live in a group home and receive training and supervision for the rest of their lives, or they may move on to more independent living. The Adult Minimal Supervision Program is basically a service for people who only lack one or two skills for living completely independently, without any staff support. The skills most commonly taught are money handling, food preparation, and transportation skills.

Family Resource Services is another major program offered in Pennsylvania. The primary aim of this program is to offer a wide variety of support services to enable parents of "mentally retarded" children to keep their children at home. As noted earlier, Family Resource Services are available to adoptive parents, foster parents and to "mentally retarded" adults living independently in the community. These services are listed below:

### Community Living Arrangement Services
Developmental maximation unit
Intensive habit shaping
Structured correctional
Child development
Adult training
Adult minimal supervision
Family relief

## Staff

The front-line staff members for our service programs must meet state civil service requirements, although they work for provider agencies or counties. Personnel are recruited through civil service bulletins, newspaper advertisements, and contacts with colleges. The starting salary for front-line staff members is approximately $6,500 per year, plus free room and board. Staff members are evaluated annually using a rating system. The typical ratio in the residential settings funded by our office is one staff member to three clients. This relatively high staffing ratio reduces staff pressure, prevents worker burn-out, promotes staff retention, and lessens operating and staff training costs.

## Costs

The costs of our services depend on the particular needs of the client. We don't fix specific costs to identifiable disabilities. We set a general range of expenditure depending on the needs of individuals. The average cost per client for services provided through our system during the 1975–1976 fiscal year was $5,940. The costs for a particular client can fluctuate dramatically from year to year. For example, in settings with a live-in nurse the cost per resident may be $45.00 per day of state monies with approximately another $3.00 per day from Supplemental Security Income (SSI). Although this service is expensive, the average cost per day for institutional services in Pennsylvania is $70.00 per day per client.

The CLA program is totally funded through state dollars, with the exception of room and board payments supplied through SSI. Program funding is awarded to provider agencies in the form of annual cash grants, paid on a quarterly basis by counties. The first quarter payment is supplied at the beginning of the fiscal year. Subsequent payments are based on monthly bills submitted by provider agencies in relation to approved, line-item expenditures.

## Comprehensiveness

One requirement for clients served through our office is that everyone must be involved in an appropriate day program or competitive employment unless they are too medically fragile to leave their living quarters or are elderly and do not wish to engage in work activity. For medically fragile children, public school teachers provide services in the home setting. The Department of Education supplies programming services during the day and the Department of Welfare provides similar services in the evenings and on weekends. Early education services, down to 2 years of age, are also available through either the Department of Education or the Department of Welfare.

Beginning in 1976, we have automatically paid 100% of the costs of vocational workshop training for clients entering CLA services for 3 years. After the third year the State pays 90% and the county 10%. This policy has greatly expanded the availability of vocational services for clients and has assured an adequate supply of day program slots.

Our office also provides transportation services for physically handicapped people who live in rural areas. Funds are made available for the lease of a vehicle on an annual basis.

We attempt to stress the use of generic services whenever possible. We generally do not need specialized dental, medical, barber, or recreational services for persons labeled "mentally retarded." Instead, we need to utilize and support existing community services to promote the greater physical and social integration of our constituency.

## LESSONS WE HAVE LEARNED

Sometimes we learn more from our mistakes than from those things we do correctly. This has certainly been our experience in attempting to develop normalized community services for Pennsylvania's citizens labeled "mentally retarded." The original continuum of community-based services that we created in Pennsylvania almost 6 years ago was patterned after the ENCOR service system. We have since made significant revisions in ENCOR's design. Today we are basically administering two types of residential settings: those for children and those for adults. As noted earlier, we also provide a variety of ancillary services, such as medical and behavior shaping services, to meet individual clients' needs in these two general settings.

### Smallness

We do not have a high proportion of clients served in group homes. We deemphasized the group home strategy early in our history. We started approximately 100 group homes and 50 apartments during our first couple of years of program development, but have only developed about 25 additional group homes during the last few years. We now primarily implement our programs in apartments or small homes housing up to three clients. Over 400 new apartment programs have been established during the past 3 years. Our group homes serve six to eight clients and our apartments serve three or fewer clients.

We believe that a smaller number of clients per setting has distinct advantages:

1.  Clients are less likely to learn inappropriate behavior from one another when the number of handicapped residents is kept low.
2.  The rate of staff burn-out is reduced with fewer clients per setting.
3.  Settings are less specialized, which reduces the need to bounce clients from one service setting to another to achieve less restrictive living arrangements.
4.  Neighbors are less likely to oppose the establishment of a residential program when three or fewer clients are served.
5.  Apartments are easier to locate and lease than larger dwellings and are more likely to be located near transportation and shopping facilities.
6.  Start-up periods are decreased for new programs because zoning regulations are not affected and renovations are not generally needed.

As an example of how our thinking has changed relative to size, we initially established three Developmental Maximation Units for groups of 20 nonambulatory, medically complex people. These units were set up in wings of hospitals or nursing homes. Recognizing the poor quality of life experienced in such settings, we next moved to three-bed units. Today we are serving many medically fragile clients in single-client placement sites.

As another example, there was a period in our early years when we were putting higher functioning children into small group homes. Today we are capable of enabling most parents to keep their mildly disabled child at home through our Family Resource Services and other support systems. We have become very careful to support, and not needlessly supplant, clients' natural homes. Properly supported, family members represent a tremendous resource to children and adults with special needs.

## Normalization

One of the major factors we tried to develop from the inception of our program was a strong commitment to normalization. We wanted to stress the importance of developing culturally acceptable behavior through using culturally appropriate intervention strategies. One of the big problems we encountered very early, however, was that program staffs often become hyperactive about PASS and normalization. They thought that normalization meant you must program every minute of the client's life: Monday night was bowling, Tuesday night was ceramics, and so on. It simply drove clients crazy! We finally convinced the staffs that one aspect of good programming is leisure periods wherein clients are allowed to just sit back and take it easy. This was a very difficult lesson for many staff members to learn.

A key ingredient related to normalization, one that can be seen particularly in settings housing three or fewer clients, is the emotional bonding that takes place between clients and staff members. In smaller, more normative settings, staff members are able to lead more typical life-styles and to relate to clients in more effective and less artificial ways. Limiting the number of clients per setting results in more verbal interaction and touching between clients and staff members, which affords all parties a much more typical life-style than the one that exists in group homes or larger settings.

## Start-up Help

As mentioned earlier, most counties purchase community services from nonprofit vendors. One of the problems that we have consistently faced is the need to encourage desirable people to establish and maintain placement sites. We now have prepared a cookbook from A to Z of the steps involved in establishing community residential services, called the *Implementation Packet: Community Living Arrangements Program for Citizens Who Are Mentally Retarded* (1). It includes our policies and regulations on community living arrangements; the roles and responsibilities of the state, regional offices, counties, and service providers; a model contract between a county and a service provider; a recommended budget system and budget standards; an application for project funding; a step-by-step procedure for developing community living arrangements in Pennsylvania; and reporting forms on vacancies, special incidents, fire reports. This is a government document. It can be mailed to you upon request at no charge.

We've also made the financial aspects of start-up much easier. A new service-providing agency getting off the ground in Pennsylvania does not need one penny, one residential setting, or one staff member. It simply fills out the application forms in our implementation packet, which are based on PASS and require an annual line-item budget for specific services, such as developmental programming, transportation, leisure time activities, clothing, and food. If the agency's application is consistent with the priorities of its county's plan and sufficient monies exist in the county's budget, the program will immediately receive 25% of its first year's funding. In other words, if the program's yearly budget is $100,000, the provider agency will receive $25,000 as the first quarterly payment so that a director can be hired and the program can get off the ground. We currently experience very little difficulty in identifying providers and in initiating services.

Human services may be funded on the basis of program allotments or on the basis of a pre-set amount per client. There are liabilities associated with both program funding and per diem funding. Under program funding providers are sometimes slow to fill residential spaces because program monies still arrive when spaces are unoccupied. Additionally, program funding generally seems to necessitate a greater amount of paperwork. Under per diem funding providers are sometimes slow to move clients who are ready to live in less restrictive settings and are economically pressured to take an inappropriate client rather than risking a loss of funds associated with waiting for a more appropriate referral.

We have opted for program funding because: 1) it gets service providers' minds off the dollar on a day-to-day basis, 2) it gives providers a set budget for the whole year at the beginning of the year so they don't face bankruptcy if they are unable to keep beds filled, and 3) it facilitates directing provider attention to service quality versus service quantity. Whatever method is chosen, it is important to have a good system for fiscal accountability and monitoring.

## Planning Ahead

One of the major problems we had in our first few years was a lack of fiscal comprehensiveness. We had all the money we needed for residential settings but failed to have sufficient fiscal coordination to support day programs for adults. Often, adult clients were left sitting at home during the last couple of months of each fiscal year because their day program money ran out. We finally corrected this problem. We now have a categorical amount that can be used for both living arrangements and day programs.

Our current fiscal planning format starts at the county level and works its way up from counties to regions to the state level. Plans are established for a 5-year time frame. The first year of any plan is very realistic, and the other 4 years are projections to be modified on a yearly basis. We have recently experienced a $7 million budget increase, the largest single budget increase for new programs in Pennsylvania, largely due to data derived from our planning process. It is a beautiful sight to behold when planning works in this fashion. Not only did we get residential monies, we also received day program monies sufficient to develop comprehensive programs for all new clients.

## Placement Stability

Our initial programs were highly specialized and required clients to move once they reached higher levels of independence. Now we are trying to stabilize clients' living situations by not moving clients around as much as we did with earlier strategies. We now move staff members and/or employ less specialized staff members who can continue with clients with temporary support from itinerant resource specialists.

## Consumer Involvement

We are highly committed to parental participation and to direct consumer involvement. We supply PASS training sessions every other month in a different section of Pennsylvania that are attended by parents, primary consumers, and staff. One major factor that we push hard is client involvement in decision making regarding their lives. We are striving from a very early age to give children opportunities to make decisions. They learn to decide what to do when they can watch *Sesame Street,* play with a range of toys, or look at pictures in a book. Learning self-control is crucial for eventual independent living.

Parents and clients should be given every opportunity to be involved in making decisions regarding policies and activities of human service agencies. Just about every service-providing agency in Pennsylvania operates a client advisory group that makes recommendations to the board of directors and/or executive director. Professionals do not have all the answers. Programs work best when a partnership exists between service-providing staffs, parents, and clients.

## Public Education

Public education is an essential feature of successful community program development. I have been involved in numerous zoning hassles and have probably learned more about people labeled "mentally retarded" in such situations than any place else. For example, did you know that if a mentally retarded person walks on one square inch of your front lawn, your whole yard dies? Or that "mentally retarded" people can't cross streets or go up and down steps? These claims were actually made. They illustrate how far we have to go in revising public attitudes and beliefs toward people with special needs. This is an enormous issue. It challenges our ingenuity and cannot be overlooked.

## Change Is Slow

It is my experience that we must be very patient and persistent in what we are trying to accomplish. Those committed to community services must sometimes wait for government bureaucrats and other societal leaders to finally fade away before significant progress can be achieved. It is hoped the people who replace them will have a better commitment to our constituency.

The intransigence of some leaders may on occasion be a blessing in disguise. Sound social service systems cannot be developed overnight. It takes time to build appropriate organizational structures, funding channels, policies, regulations, evaluation strategies, and service systems. It's not advisable to start out with the clients who are the most complex problems because they offer the greatest chance for failure. Initial success is of utmost importance. Community agencies that have never provided developmental services cannot give first-rate services overnight. You must take time to give new agencies support, direction, and experience before moving to highly difficult clients. You must take time to give the emerging system every opportunity to succeed.

When you're dealing with a population of 12 million people, as we are in Pennsylvania, you do not develop a sound community-based service system in 5 years. It obviously takes a lot longer. We have worked very hard to develop a firm undergirding for the community service system needed in Pennsylvania. We have kept our programs flexible during their emergence and as a consequence we have adopted better ways of doing some things. Most of these better ways, incidentally, have come from service providers, not from state government. If you wait for state government to identify needed service innovations, you are likely to be in big trouble. Open communication between community service providers and state government leaders is essential for constructive service advancement.

## Staff Training

It is really a tough job, in my estimation, day in and day out, to work with people who demonstrate special needs. It is imperative that we strive to keep staff skill levels high and to minimize the pressures that workers face. Staff members need training, plenty of free time, and a normative life-style. The smaller living units that we are now providing have produced a notable improvement in staff morale.

Many community service providers are people committed to helping clients change in socially desirable ways. They find it very rewarding to see clients develop independence and productivity. We must support community service agents by teaching them efficient procedures for helping clients grow and develop. We must modify rate structures to provide incentives to service providers for client advancement.

Pennsylvania provides two basic types of training for front line staffs: PASS and Project Main. PASS training sensitizes staff members to the principle of normalization. Project Main increases staff skills in the areas of individual assessment and programming. We are also engaged in developing a staff training model in conjunction with certain colleges. We are concerned with establishing a manpower development model and career ladder similar to that existing in Canada. We need to train new staff members and to retrain institutional staff members to enter community programs. We are investigating certification programs based on 2-year degrees and 4-year degrees, backed by increases in salaries and other benefits. We are on the right track but much remains to be accomplished in this area.

## Accountability

We clearly must show that clients derive benefits from our services. Our state legislature investigated our community living arrangement program 2 years ago. They indicated that we must demonstrate benefits to clients before we could expect substantial increases in program monies. We are presently engaged in a large-scale effort to do just that. We are rigorously evaluating the developmental growth of clients whose instructors receive intensive levels of staff development training. The initial data from this project are very favorable. I suspect that the tentative outcomes of this project were a major factor leading to the large budget increase that our bureau received this year.

We push for accountability in three different areas: program quality as measured by PASS, fiscal accountability as assessed through our specially designed fiscal audit system, and client outcome accountability as evaluated through individual assessments. We are concerned with generating maximum client growth in normalized settings for an economical cost.

## MAJOR PROBLEMS

Our two biggest problems are in the areas of: 1) manpower development and 2) neighborhood oversaturation. Manpower development is becoming particularly critical because of the shift that is occurring in the types of clients we are serving. During the first few years most of the client population we dealt with exhibited moderate to mild disabilities. We are now to the point that most people left in our public institutions are classified as severely or profoundly retarded. Most have serious medical and/or behavioral problems. Aside from individuals who are leaving their homes in the community, almost all of our future work will center on a highly dependent group of persons. This situation creates great demands for staff training. Curricular materials and programming strategies simply do not exist in many cases.

The issue of neighborhood oversaturation has become vexing. We work very hard to control the distances between our service settings, but we have no control over other agencies serving different special needs groups, such as juvenile corrections. The sheer number of consumers served by social welfare agencies and the limited availability of affordable housing intensify this problem. We hope to overcome this problem through increased interagency communication.

## QUESTIONS AND ANSWERS

QUESTION: What kind of feedback do you get from clients when you ask them to move from one setting to another?

KNOWLTON: We sometimes have people who do not want to move. I think there are always going to be some people who say, "Hey, I'm in an institution, I've been here 20 years and I don't want to leave." And there are others in community settings who will not want to move. With the approach we're adopting now, they don't have to move; we move staff members.

When you're talking about publicly funded living settings, it's pretty difficult to justify purchasing intensive structure and supervision for the person who no longer needs it. We must balance the desires of the client and the cost to society of satisfying his or her desires. One of the things we have to watch out for is that we operate at the economic level of the client. I've seen many group homes that were so plush, with a color TV as big as a movie screen, and things that clients will never afford at their potential earning level. We must maintain attention to conserving society's social welfare expenditures while providing high quality environments for clients.

QUESTION: How close are you on age mixing? What are your criteria for grouping people by chronological age?

KNOWLTON: For children, we have a fairly wide range. One home may have one person who is 1 year old, one who is 7, and another who is 16. We want people to see that a child moves out on his or her own after reaching a certain age. It's anticipated that when you become an adult you move away from the home setting and develop one of your own. In adult settings, we may have an age range of 18 through 30 in one setting and 30 through about 45 or 50 in another. Some individuals may fit more properly into a higher or lower age range, depending on their personality and how they get along with other people.

QUESTION: Do you provide community alternatives for everyone? That is, can you meet every individual's needs?

KNOWLTON: One of the things we try to do, but are not always successful in doing, is to provide living settings that will meet everybody's needs. I frankly don't think it's possible to meet everybody's needs. To begin with, clients very rarely know each other when they move into a program. Moreover, even when they go in as friends, they may end up as enemies after living with each other.

Many people are concerned that clients should have the right to choose, but the choices they have are so poor and their need for security is so deep. Those of us who are responsible for service development and quality of life must create a range of choices. We cannot wait! We must create apartments, train staffs, and build good programs before clients have to make unjust choices. I agree that people should have involvement in decision making about where they live. But clients' choices have little meaning in the absence of reasonable alternatives. We must offer a flexible array of service options.

## REFERENCE

1. *Implementation Packet: Community Living Arrangements Program for Citizens Who Are Mentally Retarded.* 1977. Office of Mental Retardation, Department of Public Welfare, Commonwealth of Pennsylvania, Harrisburg.

# MAKING IT WORK

## A Review of the Empirical Literature on Community Living Arrangements

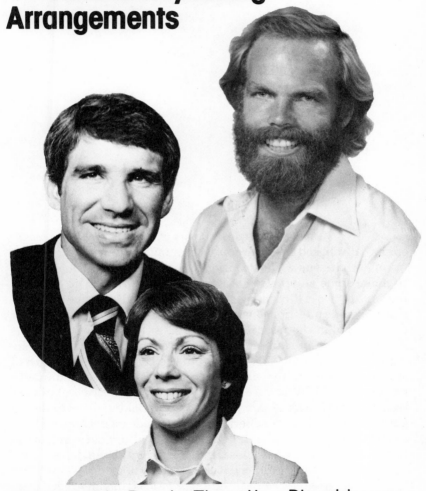

Charles A. Peck, Timothy Blackburn,
and Georgeanne White-Blackburn

*The purpose of this chapter is to survey recent* empirically based literature on community living arrangements (CLAS) for citizens with exceptional needs. The broad objective is to make some summative statements about the major research findings in two critical areas: CLA outcomes and effective CLA practices. Specific questions and issues that address these broad areas are explored in the research literature.

First of all, are individuals who enter the community remaining in the community? That is, from the perspective of length of stay in the community and readmission rates, does community placement work? What are the factors affecting success of CLAS or return to institutions? Are people in CLAS making developmental gains comparable to or superior to those made in institutional settings? Are they enjoying a better quality of life outside institutions? Essentially, what does the research say about the quantity and quality of successful client adjustment in CLAS?

Second, what are some program practices that have been demonstrated to be effective in CLAS? What service components have been successfully utilized in CLA programs? What types of developmental training for residents have been shown to be successful? What staff training procedures have proved effective?

Finally, based on existing research, what are some possible conclusions regarding program practices that seem promising for CLA settings? What priority areas are indicated for additional research and program development? What implications does the philosophical perspective of normalization have for the accomplishments and future directions of CLA research and program development?

## OUTCOMES OF COMMUNITY LIVING ARRANGEMENTS

Perhaps the most consistently pursued research questions about CLAs have focused on identifying variables associated with the successful adjustment of people re-entering the community after a period of institutionalization (1, 2, 3, 4, 5, 6). Two additional areas of CLA research that have received some attention are quality of life (7, 8, 9, 10) and developmental outcomes of CLA programs (8, 11, 12). Each of these research areas is reviewed herein.

### Successful Transition to CLAs

The overwhelming majority of CLA studies have attempted to isolate attributes of individuals with developmental special needs that are important in determining success or failure in adjusting to community living. Edgerton (13) conducted two follow-up studies of a group of people discharged from a state institution for the mentally retarded. In the earlier study, 48 people who had been living in the community for an average of 6 years were interviewed. Edgerton found that the adjustment of these individuals was generally successful, but that their success appeared to be dependent in many cases on the existence of a "benefactor." The role of the benefactor in assisting a recently deinstitutionalized person to cope with community life was suggested as more critical than any particular skill, training, or other experience the person may have had. However, in a 10-year follow-up interview with 30 of the original 48 people, Edgerton and Bercovici (2) found that the benefactor could no longer be considered the major determinant of success in community adjustment. It was also reported that vocational success did not affect community adjustment as powerfully as previously supposed. Edgerton summarized the findings of the 1967 and 1976 studies by noting that researchers have discovered very little about factors determining successful community adjustment of people labeled "mentally retarded."

Eagle (1) conducted a follow-up study of 12,471 people discharged from institutions. He found that 39.6% of these people were later readmitted. Analyzing reasons cited for the readmissions, Eagle found that anti-social actions, undesirable personal conduct, health problems, and adverse environmental factors were the most common problems. Adverse environmental factors (lack of support from family or caregivers, economic problems, community objections, illness of caregivers, or closing of the CLA facility) were cited in one-third of the readmissions. Eagle cautioned that, in many instances, these data were based on social worker evaluations of the reasons for CLA failures and are therefore somewhat inconclusive. He emphasized that the results of this study and others in the existing literature have not successfully identified predictive criteria for community adjustment.

Reviewing studies completed several years after Eagle (1) and Edgerton (13), apparent consensus has still not been achieved regarding which factors are predictive of a handicapped individual's success or failure in a CLA. However, some broad similarities along the dimensions of adaptive social behavior and health problems can be seen in the results of several recent studies. Sternlicht (14), in a review of the literature on problems of people in CLAS, found that unacceptable behavior and poor health of the residents were the most consistently cited variables in CLA failure. Support for these findings is provided by Pagel and Whitling (5), who conducted a follow-up of 117 deinstitutionalized people placed in CLAS and found that "maladaptive" behavior (behaviors unacceptable to caregivers) and health problems were the most frequent causes of an individual's failure to succeed in the living arrangement. Behavior problems were also cited by Eyman and Call (3) as a major block to the deinstitutionalization process. Nihira and Nihira (15) taped interviews with 109 caregivers responsible for 424 people with developmental special needs. They found that 86.7% of the incidents recalled by the caregivers that jeopardized the health, general, or legal welfare of the residents involved problems with conduct or emotional disturbance as opposed to skill deficiencies.

A follow-up study of 440 people who moved to the community conducted by Gollay (16) showed that one of the most commonly cited CLA problems was family relationship conflicts. The other most common problem was finding and keeping a job. In contrast to other studies, Gollay noted that medical needs and socially unacceptable behavior were rated by caregivers as among the least problematic areas of CLA service delivery. Conflicting data on the need for improved medical service have also been reported by O'Conner (17). Surveying the questionnaire responses of 611 family care operators, O'Conner found that 89% rated medical services to their residents as adequate or very adequate.

In summary, research efforts to identify factors affecting CLA success or failure have not yielded clearly interpretable results. Two factors have consistently reappeared in the literature. Social behavior adjustment is the variable most often cited as critical to an individual's success in a CLA (1, 3, 5, 14, 15, 16). Health problems are also cited by several researchers as the reason for CLA failure (1, 5, 14), although data also exist that do not support health problems as a cause of CLA failure (16, 17). Although the data describing the role of social behavior and health problems in influencing success or failure in CLAs are incomplete, they nevertheless mandate increased program development and research effort in these areas.

## Quality of Life in CLAs

Issues relating to the quality of services delivered in CLAs and institutional settings and the quality of life enjoyed by residents have received considerable attention in recent literature (7, 8, 9, 10, 18). Central to interest in these issues is the recognition that simply remaining in the community is not a sufficiently rigorous criterion of CLA success (2). Several studies have attempted to compare the quality of services and resulting quality of life across various residential settings. In a review of the literature, Balla (7) attempted to assess the relationship of institutional size to quality of care. Four dimensions of care were investigated: a) resident care practices, b) behavioral functioning, c) discharge rates, and d) parental and community involvement. Balla found differences in resident care practices favoring smaller residential settings, but smallness did not in itself ensure quality of resident care practices. Balla also cited evidence indicating that people placed in CLAs had more contact with their family and the community than people in institutions. No conclusive data were available on differences in behavioral functioning or discharge rates related to institutional size.

In a study of large programs (30–50 residents) and small programs (4–6 residents), Bjaanes and Butler (8) assessed the attitudinal, supportive, physical, and behavioral components of the residential environments. They found that *larger* settings, which were board and care facilities, more closely approximated the ideals of normalization than did the smaller home care facilities. Additionally, more independent behavior was observed in the larger residential settings. However, their investigation was carried out with only two facilities of each type, thus raising serious questions about the generality of the study.

McCormick, Balla, and Zigler (9) compared residential services in the United States and Scandinavia and found that differences in care practices correlated with size of the residential facility. Residential care practices were evaluated as more institution oriented in large facilities and more resident oriented in smaller facilities. Care practices were assessed by rigidity of routine, regimentation, depersonalization, and extent of staff-resident interaction. Scheerenberger (10) took a somewhat different approach to assessing quality of care in CLAS by interviewing 75 formerly institutionalized persons in the state of Wisconsin to obtain information on normalization practices and consumer satisfaction. He found that consumers were generally quite satisfied with CLA services and most satisfied in the smaller settings. The procedure of obtaining consumer ratings as quality of life measures has also been suggested by Edgerton and Bercovici (2). This seems a particularly appropriate suggestion regarding this line of research.

While a strong case has certainly been made in support of the superior quality of life offered by CLAS (17, 19, 20), evidence remains that simply living in the community does not in itself ensure a specific quality of life (2, 7). Size of the community residential setting does not seem to be an adequate predictor of the quality of CLA life in all cases (7, 8). It seems clear that professionals who assist persons to move into the community must take responsibility for rigorously evaluating the quality of life in CLAS rather than assuming that community placement per se is adequate. Although size is certainly a relevant factor, other dimensions of importance include quality of developmental programming (17), availability of support services (18), quality of residents' interactions with staff (8), and consumer satisfaction (10).

## Developmental Outcomes of CLA Programming

It has been amply demonstrated that the direction of residential services for individuals with developmental special needs has been innocent of empirical guidance (20). This is strikingly evident when one reviews the investigations of developmental progress made by people in CLAs. Although there have been few studies that directly investigated developmental outcomes in CLAs, there clearly is agreement on the importance and value of such research (8, 9, 16, 21).

A notable instance of well-designed research investigating developmental gains in CLAS was reported by Close (11). He studied increases in skills made on criterion-referenced measures by eight CLA residents and seven matched institutionalized residents. All participants were labeled severely or profoundly retarded. Comparing gains made across a 1-year period, Close found that the CLA residents acquired more self-help and social skills than the institutionalized people. Although this study demonstrated the exciting possibilities of CLA programming, it cannot be viewed as representative of typical CLA settings. The residential facility in this study enjoyed the benefits of close association with an academic center of reputed excellence in the area of developmental services. Rich staffing ratios, sophisticated developmental programming, and expert supervision are certainly not common attributes of CLAs at present.

Another comparison of developmental progress of institutionalized and deinstitutionalized people was conducted by Schroeder and Henes (12). They made a matched-control comparison of 19 institutionalized people and 19 people residing in four group homes in the community. Results indicated that developmental gains, as measured by the Progress Assessment Chart, were greater for the CLA group than the institutionalized group. However, the authors noted that normalization practices, as indicated by PASS (20) ratings, were not always correlated with developmental gains.

Taken together, these studies provide tentative support for the efficacy of developmental programming in CLAS. The extremely small number of residences studied, however, may restrict the generality of the results. Also, McCormick et al. (9) have noted that a wide variance in developmental progress has been reported for individuals in institutional settings. Additional work, as exemplified by Close (11) and Schroeder and Henes (12), is needed before definitive statements can be made about developmental outcomes of CLA programming.

## Summary of CLA Outcome Research

The empirical literature on CLA outcomes may be divided into: a) studies of factors affecting successful adjustment to CLAS, b) studies of quality of life, and c) studies of developmental gains. Literature on adjustment factors suggested that social behavior problems and medical problems may often affect success in CLAS. As noted earlier, most of the research on success in CLAS has been focused on characteristics of the resident. It appears that identification of variables predictive of success should involve increased attention to the characteristics of community settings and the characteristics of releasing institutions.

The quality of life literature provided support for the widely held opinion that CLAS are more pleasant places to live in than institutions (7, 9, 10, 18). Care practices were found to be more resident oriented in smaller residential settings (7, 9). However, an important finding was that size did not *always* correlate with quality of care (7, 8).

Research on developmental gains in CLA settings was difficult to locate. Two recent studies, however, indicated that superior developmental progress was made by individuals residing in the community as opposed to institutions (11, 12). These reports provide only tentative findings in this important area of research.

Unfortunately, the empirical literature on CLA outcomes has not been characterized by cohesive lines of well-conceived and thorough research (4, 6, 8, 21). Several reasons for the inadequacy of existing research on factors affecting CLA outcomes have been suggested. The complexity and number of possible variables involved in CLA success have made research in this area quite difficult (1, 2, 6). However, factors limiting the generality and validity of most completed studies are based on much more than methodological difficulties. Characteristics of the receiving CLA and the releasing institution have been largely ignored. Thus, potentially critical issues associated with preparatory training within the institution as well as the accommodative capacity of the CLA have not been investigated.

The expansion of the CLA movement has been one of the most vigorous responses to the ideological principles of normalization (22). However, the foregoing view of the empirical literature makes it obvious that we do not yet know how to consistently ensure successful adjustment, quality of life, or developmental gains in CLAs. An alarming corollary to the increase in releases from institutions in recent years has been an equally dramatic increase in readmissions (22, 23). Thus, it is apparent that, despite available models of effective CLA programming (such as those described in this volume), a disturbing number of residential programs are failing to adequately support people with developmental special needs in the community. It seems imperative that increased attention be accorded research efforts to develop and empirically validate improved methods of delivering CLA services. The next section of this chapter describes some empirically demonstrated program practices relevant to community residential settings that have been reported to date.

## DEMONSTRATED CLA PROGRAM PRACTICES

Although critical variables affecting the success of community living arrangements have not been identified, several dimensions of program development have been emphasized for their possible value in improving CLA services. First, provision of appropriate and effective developmental intervention is suggested as integral to high quality CLA programming by several reviewers (8, 11, 17, 24). Staff training is another program dimension that seems of obvious importance to developing high quality CLAs (17, 24, 25). The importance of educational, recreational, and vocational training has also been emphasized by some investigators (1, 17, 26, 27, 28). Each of these components of CLA service delivery is discussed briefly, and relevant examples of empirically demonstrated program practices are described.

### Developmental Intervention

Procedures for effective developmental programming in a variety of settings have been well documented in the literature (29, 30, 31, 32). A few examples of developmental intervention procedures have also been demonstrated in CLA settings. Barry, Apolloni, and Cooke (33) reported on an effective intervention package for increasing personal grooming skills of persons living in semi-independent apartment settings. They utilized contingency contracting techniques to achieve increases in behaviors like using deodorant, brushing hair, and washing, which generalized outside of direct training sessions. Robinson-Wilson (34) reported successful use of a pictorial recipe program to teach persons labeled severely retarded to cook simple foods in a CLA setting. She showed that generalized recipe following skills were increased substantially for all participants in the program.

While there are comparatively few demonstrations of developmental training programs reported from CLA settings, many procedures for teaching skills necessary for community independence have been validated with similar clients in other settings (35). For example, Bellamy and Buttars (36) used a systematic procedure to teach money counting skills to five adolescents labeled "moderately retarded" or "emotionally disturbed." All of these individuals learned to count out change to $1 and generalized this skill to noninstructional settings. In a similar study, Lowe and Cuvo (37) taught four mildly and moderately retarded persons to sum the value of coin combinations using a modeling strategy.

Transportation skills are also important to independence in the community. Page, Iwata, and Neef (38) taught five people labeled "retarded" several basic pedestrian skills. Although training was originally conducted in a classroom, generalization to actual city traffic conditions was achieved successfully. Using public transportation has been suggested necessary for community independence and successful employment (15, 39, 40, 41). In a study by Neef, Iwata, and Page (42), bus riding skills (locating, signaling, boarding, riding, and exiting a bus) were taught using both in vivo and classroom instruction. The results indicated that students in the program exhibited appropriate bus riding skills up to 12 months following training.

An important area of developmental training for individuals living in CLAS involves leisure skills. Bjaanes and Butler (8) found that residents living in four group homes spent only 3% of their free time in structured, goal-directed leisure behaviors. The remaining free time was spent in more passive activities, such as napping and watching television. These findings are supported by Gollay (16), who also reported on the typically passive use of leisure time in CLAS. Johnson and Bailey (43) successfully used a systematic developmental training procedure to increase the leisure behavior of 14 mentally retarded women living in a halfway house. Instructions, availability of materials, and prizes were shown to increase several leisure activities (e.g., playing cards, weaving, hooking rugs). The importance of the study, as the authors state, is not the specific behaviors increased, but the demonstration of the relevance of systematic instructional technology to the area of leisure behavior. Curricula have been devised for teaching leisure skills to persons with disabilities (26, 44). Data reported by Day and Day (26) show that 38% of leisure skills for which programming was attempted were successfully taught in a 2-month time period. The authors stated that the leisure skills generalized after instruction terminated, although no data were presented on this.

It is important to recognize that some characteristics are shared by these examples of successful developmental intervention. These may be categorized as systematic assessment, highly structured intervention, and rigorous evaluation of intervention outcomes. The foregoing investigations support the notion of Luckey and Addison (24) and O'Conner (17) that systematic developmental intervention, which has been demonstrated as powerfully effective in other instructional settings (30, 31, 32), may be an important component of programmatic success in CLAS.

## Staff Training

Reviewers of CLA service delivery systems have agreed on the need for greatly increased staff training efforts (5, 9, 17, 24). Although staff training procedures have been successfully developed and implemented in many developmental service settings, few empirical demonstrations of effective training for community residential staffs have been completed. In one CLA-based study, Schinke and Wong (25) investigated a training program in behavior modification techniques for group home staff persons. They reported increases in theoretical knowledge of behavior principles, job satisfaction, positive perceptions of client abilities, and use of correct training behaviors by workshop participants.

Although it has been amply demonstrated that developmental personnel can be taught to engage in appropriate training behaviors (45, 46), there has been little verification of the impact of this training on the developmental progress of the client (24). Without these types of data, difficult as they are to collect, the relative value of various staff training efforts is difficult to assess. Moreover, without a client outcome data base, we truly have no means of really knowing what competencies staff members most need in order to maximize developmental gains. It may, in fact, be that CLA staff persons will have to assume many responsibilities for daily programming of a specialized nature that have formerly been the province of professional interdisciplinary teams.

However, a few recent studies have demonstrated techniques for evaluating staff training on the basis of client progress (45, 46). For example, Fabry and Reid (45) assessed the developmental gains made by children labeled severely retarded as a measure of the effectiveness of a training program for their foster grandparents. Similarly, Koegel, Russo, and Rincover (46) evaluated a teacher training program partially by its demonstrated effects on targeted behavior of children designated as autistic. Another strategy for validating staff training outcomes has been reported by Wolf (47). He suggested that subjective measures of consumer satisfaction may offer a means of assessing the social significance of training outcomes not always provided by direct observational methodology.

## Vocational Training

The role of vocational training in ensuring CLA success has been emphasized by several investigators (16, 27, 48). A number of factors have led to a large increase in the quantity and quality of vocational training services available to persons with developmental special needs (49). Legislative support for specialized vocational training programs has greatly increased (e.g., Vocational Education Act, 1968; Developmental Disabilities Services and Facilities Construction Act, 1970; Vocational Rehabilitation Act, 1973; and the Education for All Handicapped Children Act, 1975). Particularly relevant to effective service delivery in community settings has been the development of new systematic procedures for conducting vocational training and placement for individuals with exceptional needs.

Task analysis (50, 51) has been employed with excellent results in vocational training programs. Gold (51) employed task analysis methods to teach severely and profoundly retarded persons to complete complex assembly tasks unassisted. Bellamy, Peterson, and Close (52) also reported successful training of severely and profoundly retarded persons on assembly tasks using task analysis methods. Cuvo, Leaf, and Borakove (53) task analyzed janitorial skills in a successful training program for adolescents labeled moderately retarded. In a vocational training program designed as a component to the deinstitutionalization process, Andriano (27) used task analysis and behavioral teaching strategies to train five individuals labeled severely retarded to do packaging, sorting, and collating work as Red Cross volunteers.

Many improvements in vocational training programs have focused on increasing the correspondence between training activities and jobs available in the community. A method for defining the skills critical to success on a prospective job site was developed by Belmore and Brown (54). These authors described a systematic job inventory that directs detailed attention to assessment of: a) general background information on the job, b) specific skills required to perform the job, and c) skills peripheral to the actual job but tangentially related to success. Another example of systematic assessment of critical job skills was reported by Mithaug, Hagmeier, and Haring (55). They emphasized the importance of conducting vocational training activities directly based on the characteristics of available jobs as described by their job supervisors. They noted that different supervisors did not agree on what skills are necessary for success on the job. This observation supports the importance of individualized vocational training based on differing supervisorial criteria.

## Summary of CLA Program Practices

The relatively limited body of empirical literature on CLA program practices does not presently allow conclusive programmatic recommendations. However, based on the few studies available, and extrapolations from other relevant literature, some tentative statements may be made. In the area of developmental programming, systematic approaches to assessment, intervention, and evaluation were characteristic of successful training procedures. The area of staff training, although recognized as extremely important, has not been accorded much attention in the empirical literature. It was suggested that outcomes of staff training efforts might best be evaluated in CLAs in terms of their impact on client gains. Community vocational training program practices were characterized by the use of task analysis to teach complex job skills and the systematic use of job assessment procedures to aid in defining training activities.

## NEW PERSPECTIVES ON
## RESEARCH AND PROGRAM DEVELOPMENT

After appraising the empirical literature presented in this chapter, one may have the impression that the CLA-normalization movement, as articulated so well in this volume, has proceeded independent of a data base on deinstitutionalization outcomes. CLA program development should, after all, be directly guided by the results of research on outcomes of programs aimed at deinstitutionalizing people with developmental special skills, right? Research should focus on identifying those skills crucial to success in CLAS and on procedures for teaching them, right? Wrong!

Wrong because these questions focus upon how to make the process of deinstitutionalization work—not upon how to accomplish the goals of normalization in the context of CLAS. This might be an academic distinction if it were not based on an even more crucial distinction, which has important practical and philosophical implications for research and development efforts. The distinction is between deinstitutionalization and normalization.

Central to the deinstitutionalization movement, as evidenced by the literature reviewed in this chapter, is the notion that people with special needs should be living in the community, *but* that they at present lack certain skills necessary for succeeding in the community (16, 22). Failure in CLAS is attributed to the client's lack of necessary appropriate behavior or the CLA's inability to teach that behavior (1, 3, 5, 15, 16, 20, 23, 39). In either case the reason for failure is viewed as the client's unacceptable deviance from community behavioral standards. The prescriptive solution to the problem is client training, staff training, a continuum of residential services, additional support services, or some other action taken to reduce original deviance. This is simply a new version of the old isolate, fix, and return paradigm—the medical hospitalization model. The data on rates of readmission to institutions (22, 23) tell us this model is not working well. Indeed, should we be surprised that we have not successfully taught deinstitutionalized people to demonstrate the behaviors crucial to CLA success when we have not even been able to identify those behaviors? (1, 2, 6) Viewed in this perspective, it seems somewhat indefensible to insist that individuals earn admission to CLAS by demonstrating "entry criteria." As long as people with developmental special needs are viewed as deviant from community behavioral standards, as has been the case within the deinstitutionalization movement, research and program development efforts will continue to focus on ways of ameliorating the deviance—ways to make people acceptable.

If, in contrast, one views developmental differences simply as differences (amplifications of the same types of differences we accept every day), then research and program development are no longer encumbered with the primary and unmanageable responsibility of making differences disappear! Rather, efforts may be directed toward fostering the integration and participation of persons with developmental special needs in community life regardless of differences. This is the heart, if not the cited definition, of normalization. Research and program development for client and staff training are not discarded, but the evaluation of their efficacy is made in terms of increased independence, participation, and integration in the community rather than attainment of developmental criteria of questionable validity. Responsibility for achieving the goals of deinstitutionalization has rested with the clients and trainers (in institutions and CLAs), that is, to reduce, as much as possible, the client's deviance from behavioral norms. However, the responsibility for achieving the goals of normalization rests on substantially broader shoulders. Certainly the client and the trainer must continue to work toward attainment of skills related to independence in community living. But the CLA and the community have a much-expanded responsibility to ensure integration and participation in community life for all individuals, regardless of developmental status. As they have in other civil rights movements (e.g., minority and women's rights), social service agencies and the community at large must make vigorous efforts to achieve the goals of social reform. Research and program development should play an important role in shaping these efforts.

Research on ways in which CLAs can facilitate independence, integration, and participation in the community may begin on the familiar turf of client and staff training. However, training efforts will be evaluated in terms of how well they assist in achieving the goals of normalization rather than only in terms of how well they reduce developmental differences. For example, criteria for successful skill training must include assessment of whether the client uses the skill as appropriately and independently as possible in the community. Staff training, in turn, should be evaluated in terms of increases in client skills demonstrated in the community. Setting performance criteria and prioritizing targets for skill training might be guided by normative data collected on the behavioral ecology of the community.

Further research needs to be conducted to identify characteristics of CLAS that successfully serve highly dependent clients. Similarly, characteristics of the community at large that facilitate integration and participation—highly dependent individuals—in community life must be investigated. A particularly promising line of research and program development, and one that has received some attention in the literature, is the expansion of generic resource agencies to serve all people on the basis of need.

Traditionally, certain categories of people have been excluded or accorded limited service by generic agencies. Ex-convicts, the elderly, and minority groups have found such exclusion. For some groups, particularly the developmentally disabled, use of generic resources has been made contingent upon meeting certain entry criteria *besides* need for the service. Even when extraneous entry criteria are removed (e.g., providing wheelchair ramps to public buildings) the de facto non-use of the agency shows that the access provided is only token. It is analogous to the removal of poll taxes and voter literacy tests in the 1960s: minority groups still did not fully *use* the franchise. It is clear that access is not enough. Research and program development efforts must take affirmative action to discover ways of ensuring that generic service delivery is extended to all people on the basis of need—including individuals with special needs.

Some examples of ways to ensure that individuals with special developmental needs participate in generic service benefits have been reported in the CLA literature. Corcoran and French (28) investigated a method of integrating adults with special developmental needs into community recreational activities. These adults enrolled in a state college course designated to teach the specific recreational skills involved in utilizing recreational facilities at the college and in the community. Physical education majors were assigned as proctors for the course, and provided one-to-one instruction in each necessary skill. The instruction successfully allowed some individuals to independently participate in community recreational activities and provided the necessary support to ensure that every individual was able to make use of the generic recreational services to some extent.

Another possible way to facilitate integration and participation in generic service benefits was described by Fox and Karan

(56). They reported on the successful use of a liaison person to assist people with developmental special needs in transition to CLAS. Referral to appropriate generic service agencies and implementation of training programs to assure maximum transfer of skills to the community settings were important responsibilities of the liaison person.

Although specific training in the use of generic resources will doubtless be an important focus of research on methods of attaining the goals of normalization, an equally important area for investigation is the expansion of the commitment by generic service agencies and the community at large to these goals. This might include removing de facto restrictions on use of community resources (e.g., removing "special" schedules for people with developmental special needs to use recreational facilities). It might mean retaining some restrictions, but clearly defining them in terms of obvious necessity (e.g., all individuals who use a pool must be continent). Evaluation of new services for people with developmental special needs may be done in the context of how the service might be delivered by or within the framework of existing generic agencies or community support systems (e.g., sex education might be provided for *all* people by Planned Parenthood agencies).

In summary, our review of the empirical literature has made it absolutely clear that we have not yet satisfactorily defined effective and reliable methods for achieving success in CLA programming (22, 23). Methodological inadequacies represent only tangential problems. More important is the possibility that research and program development efforts have been largely directed toward the wrong goal: making deinstitutionalization work. Implicit in this goal is a definition of the individual with developmental special needs as deviant from accepted behavior standards. Rather than attempting to remediate the perceived deviance, it is suggested that future research and program development efforts be directed toward achieving the goals of normalization: independence, participation, and integration into the community, developmental differences notwithstanding. It is necessary that research and program development be guided by the recognition that token access to the community is not enough. Methods must be found to actualize the notion that generic service agencies, and the general community, have an obligation to respond with equal vigor to the fundamentally "special" needs of all people.

## REFERENCES

1. Eagle, E. 1967. Prognosis and outcome of community placement of institutionalized retardates. Am. J. Ment. Def. 72:232–243.
2. Edgerton, R., and Bercovici, S. 1976. The cloak of competence: Years later. Am. J. Ment. Def. 80:485–497.
3. Eyman, R. K., and Call, T. 1977. Maladaptive behavior and community placement of mentally retarded persons. Am. J. Ment. Def. 82:137–144.
4. McCarver, R., and Craig, E. 1974. Placement of the retarded in the community: Prognosis and outcome. In N. R. Ellis (Ed.), International Review of Research in Mental Retardation, Volume 7. Academic Press, Inc., New York.
5. Pagel, S. E., and Whitling, C. A. 1978. Readmissions to a state hospital for mentally retarded persons: Reasons for community placement failure. Ment. Retard. 16:164–166.
6. Rosen, M., Floor, L., and Baxter, D. 1972. Prediction of community adjustment: A failure at cross validation. Am. J. Ment. Def. 77:111–112.
7. Balla, D. 1976. Relationship of institution size to quality of care: A review of the literature. Am. J. Ment. Def. 81:117–124.
8. Bjaanes, A., and Butler, E. 1974. Environmental variation in community care facilities for mentally retarded persons. Am. J. Ment. Def. 78:429–439.
9. McCormick, M., Balla, D., and Zigler, E. 1975. Resident care practices in institutions for retarded persons: A cross institutional, cross-cultural study. Am. J. Ment. Def. 80:1–17.
10. Scheerenberger, R. C. 1977. Community settings for mentally retarded persons: Satisfaction and activities. Ment. Retard. 15(4):3–7.
11. Close, D. 1977. Community living for severely and profoundly retarded adults: A group home study. Educ. Train. Ment. Retard. 12:256–262.
12. Schroeder, S. R., and Henes, C. 1978. Assessment of progress of institutionalized and deinstitutionalized retarded adults: A matched-control comparison. Ment. Retard. 16:147–148.
13. Edgerton, R. 1967. The Cloak of Competence: Stigma in the Lives of the Mentally Retarded. University of California Press, Berkeley.
14. Sternlicht, M. 1978. Variables affecting foster care placement of institutionalized retarded residents. Ment. Retard. 16:25–28.
15. Nihira, L., and Nihira, K. 1977. Jeopardy in community placement. Am. J. Ment. Def. 79:538–544.
16. Gollay, E. 1977. Deinstitutionalized mentally retarded people: A closer look. Educ. Train. Ment. Retard. 12:137–144.
17. O'Conner, G. 1976. Home is a good place. Monogr. Am. J. Ment. Def. 2.
18. Baker, B., Seltzer, G., and Seltzer, M. 1977. As Close as Possible. Little, Brown, & Co., Boston.

19. Blatt, B., and Kaplan, F. 1966. Christmas in Purgatory. Allyn & Bacon, Boston.
20. Wolfsensberger, W. 1976. The origin and nature of our institutional models. In R. Kugel and A. Shearer (Eds.), Changing Patterns in Residential Services for the Mentally Retarded. President's Committee on Mental Retardation, Washington, D.C.
21. Kraus, J. 1972. Supervised living in the community, and residential and employment stability of retarded male juveniles. Am. J. Ment. Def. 77:283–290.
22. Butterfield, E. 1976. Some basic changes in residential facilities. In R. Kugel and A. Shearer (Eds.), Changing Patterns in Residential Services for the Mentally Retarded. President's Committee on Mental Retardation, Washington, D.C.
23. Conroy, J. W. 1977. Trends in deinstitutionalization of the mentally retarded. Ment. Retard. 15:42–46.
24. Luckey, R. E., and Addison, M. R. 1974. Future directions in residential services: Reaction or evaluation? Train. School Bull. 71:93–100.
25. Schinke, S., and Wong, S. 1977. Evaluation of staff training in group homes for retarded persons. Am. J. Ment. Def. 82:130–136.
26. Day, R., and Day, M. 1977. Leisure skills instruction for the moderately and severely retarded: A demonstration program. Educ. Train. Ment. Retard. 12:128–131.
27. Andriano, T. A. 1977. The volunteer model of vocational habilitation as a component of the deinstitutionalization process. Ment. Retard. 15:58–61.
28. Corcoran, E., and French, R. 1977. Leisure activity for the retarded adult in the community. Ment. Retard. 15:21–23.
29. Hall, R. V. 1972. Managing Behavior. Edmark Associates, Bellevue, Wash.
30. Haring, N., and Brickler, D. (Eds.). 1978. Teaching the Severely Handicapped, Vol. III. Special Press, Columbus, Oh.
31. O'Leary, K., and O'Leary, S. (Eds.). 1972. Classroom Management. Pergamon Press, New York.
32. Snell, M. (Ed.). 1978. Systematic Instruction of the Moderately and Severely Handicapped. Charles E. Merrill Publishing Co., Columbus, Oh.
33. Barry, K., Apolloni, T., and Cooke, T. 1977. Improving the personal hygiene of mildly retarded men in a community-based residential training program. Corrective Soc. Psychiatry 23:65–68.
34. Robinson-Wilson, M. 1977. Picture recipe cards as an approach to teaching retarded adults to cook. Educ. Train. Ment. Retard. 12:69–73.
35. Adams, P., Apolloni, T., Cooke, T. P., Palyo, B., Raver, S., and Sabbag, D. (Eds.). 1978. Sonoma Developmental Curriculum. Human Services Associates, Santa Rosa, Cal.
36. Bellamy, T., and Buttars, K. L. 1975. Teaching trainable level retarded students to count money: Toward personalized in-

dependence through academic instruction. Ed. Train. Ment. Retard. 10:18–26.

37. Lowe, M., and Cuvo, A. J. 1976. Teaching coin summation to the mentally retarded. J. Appl. Behav. Anal. 9:483–489.

38. Page, T. J., Iwata, B. A., and Neef, N. A. 1976. Teaching pedestrian skills to retarded persons: Generalization from the classroom to natural environment. J. Appl. Behav. Anal. 9:433–444.

39. Nihira, L., and Nihira, K. 1975. Normalized behavior in community placement. Ment. Retard. 13:9–13.

40. Eagan, R. 1967. Should the educable mentally retarded receive driver education? Except. Child. 33:323–324.

41. Egg, M. 1965. The Different Child Grows Up. John Day, New York.

42. Neef, N. A., Iwata, B. A., and Page, T. J. 1978. Public transportation training: In vivo versus classroom instruction. J. Appl. Behav. Anal. 11:331–344.

43. Johnson, M. S., and Bailey, J. S. 1977. The modification of leisure behavior in a half-way house for retarded women. J. Appl. Behav. Anal. 10:273–282.

44. Westaway, A., and Apolloni, T. 1978. Becoming Independent: A Living Skills System. Edmark Associates, Bellevue, Wash.

45. Fabry, P., and Reid, D. 1978. Teaching foster grandparents to train severely handicapped persons. J. Appl. Behav. Anal. 11:111–123.

46. Koegel, R., Russo, D., and Rincover, A. 1977. Assessing and training teachers in the generalized use of behavior modification with autistic children. J. Appl. Behav. Anal. 10:197–205.

47. Wolf, M. M. 1978. Social validity: The case for subjective measurement or how applied behavior analysis is finding its heart. J. Appl. Behav. Anal. 11:203–214.

48. Miller, G. 1974. An on-campus community living center for the mentally retarded. Train. School Bull. 71:112–118.

49. Flexer, R., and Martin, A. 1978. Sheltered workshops and vocational training settings. In M. Snell (Ed.), Systematic Instruction of the Moderately and Severely Handicapped. Charles Merrill Publishing Co., Columbus.

50. Gold, M. 1972. Stimulus factors in skill training on a complex assembly task: Acquisition, transfer, and retention. Am. J. Ment. Def. 76:517–526.

51. Gold, M. 1976. Task analysis of a complex assembly task by the retarded blind. Except. Child. 43:78–84.

52. Bellamy, G. T., Peterson, L., and Close, D. 1975. Habilitation of the severely and profoundly retarded: Illustrations of competence. Educ. Train. Ment. Retard. 10:174–186.

53. Cuvo, A., Leaf, R., and Borakove, L. 1978. Teaching janitorial skills to the mentally retarded: Acquisition, generalization, maintenance. J. Appl. Behav. Anal. 11:345–355.

54. Belmore, K., and Brown, L. 1976. A job inventory strategy for use with severely handicapped potential workers. Madison's Alternative for Zero Exclusion. Madison Public Schools, Madison, Wisc.

55. Mithaug, D. E., Hagmeier, L. D., and Haring, N. G. 1977. The relationship between training activities and job placement in vocational education of the severely and profoundly handicapped. Am. Assoc. Educ. Sev. Profound. Hand. Rev. 2:25–45.
56. Fox, R., and Karan, O. 1976. Deinstitutionalization as a function of interagency planning: A case study. Educ. Train. Ment. Retard. 11: 255–260.

# CANADIAN DEVELOPMENTS

## Past, Present, and Direction

G. Allan Roeher

## GENERAL BACKGROUND OF
## UNITED STATES-CANADIAN DEVELOPMENTS

*In Canada and the United States trends in* human service programs of this century have been guided primarily by social bias and pragmatic considerations rather than ideology that recognized handicapped persons as equal citizens. With the advent of industrialization and urbanization, families found it increasingly difficult to cope independently with handicapped persons who grew up as ongoing dependents. A practical solution to the dilemma took the direction of development of special facilities to house such dependents. The decision to build "institutions" was necessitated by the fact that agencies serving the "normal" population were not prepared to accommodate people with special needs.

Gradual evolution of special education concepts in the 1930s and 1940s, together with post-World War II developments in physical rehabilitation for war- and industry-injured individuals, raised interest in some parents to search for additional help for their mentally handicapped children. Initially this tended to focus on some form of family relief and day activity for the child (in contrast to the present emphasis on personal development). The subsequent realization that these children benefited and developed in response to structured programming gave the pioneer parents the impetus to reach further.

With aid from limited but dedicated professional support the parent movement flourished, and the concept of a broader range of community services evolved. In contrast to many other citizen action groups that develop to stimulate others to correct a problem or assume responsibility, these parent-oriented groups assumed both self-help and advocacy functions. Because existing agencies were unwilling or unable to deliver the needed services, local associations established themselves as legally incorporated local service operating entities from the start in order to demonstrate that assistance could be delivered successfully.

By the late 1960s, services at the community level were quite extensive. With the basic "day services" then available, most families were willing and able to care for their retarded member. Still, in the minds of every parent lingered the pressing question of what would happen when they were gone or no longer able to be responsible for their offspring. A deep concern for future security, along with higher expectations of potential growth through more and better services, became the basis for seeking an even wider range of community services. Parents needed comprehensive services with continuity and assurance for safe and secure futures for their children in the community. Otherwise, when the necessity arose, institutions remained the only other alternative for assuming full and life-long responsibility.

The impact of the evolving "equal rights" and "normalization" climate is currently motivating a growing number of people to develop more innovative approaches to problem solving on these issues. These concepts have altered the posture of parents from one of hope to one of demand. In spite of the many improvements and increases in services resulting from the implementation of these precepts, many individuals are still being served either inadequately, inappropriately, or not at all.

## The United States

The U.S. Department of Health, Education and Welfare (HEW) estimates that about 6 million persons in the United States are mentally retarded, with 95% of those being mildly or moderately and

5% severely or profoundly retarded. The estimated annual cost of care and treatment for the mentally retarded in 1974 was between $8.5 and $9 billion.

In 1963, under President John F. Kennedy's influence, the improvement and expansion of community facilities and programs became a national goal. Emphasis was placed on care and treatment in the community rather than in institutions. Massive funding became available to state governments, private voluntary organizations, and universities to construct facilities, expand educational and vocational services, and provide income (pensions and/or supplemental income security), to enable mentally retarded persons to live and be served in their communities. Research and development activity, special education, human service staff training, and expansion of activity by voluntary and public agencies all benefited from a period of unparalleled growth.

At present, nearly every type of service needed by the handicapped population can be funded wholly or in part with federal monies. Well over 100 federal programs operated by 11 major departments and agencies impact either directly or indirectly on programs to serve mentally retarded persons. Income support payments are generally provided directly to individuals or through grants to state governments to cover part of the cost of services. Services tend to be uneven because of the variance in service commitment among the different states and the difference in eligibility requirements (age, income, degree of disability). There is reason to believe that the problem is not directly related to overall inadequacy of the service delivery system, but rather to inadequate use of fiscal and other resources.

With the monumental, broad-based surge of support from President Kennedy's administration, hopes were understandably high for major progress in the field. President Richard Nixon further enhanced President Kennedy's precedent, in November, 1971, by proclaiming the return of one-third of the over 200,000 mentally retarded persons in public institutions (of which 30,600 were still in state mental institutions) to useful lives in the community. In October, 1975, President Gerald Ford lent his support to the 1971 goal.

United States' courts have tended to accept the newer concepts of normalization and the right of an individual to appropriate levels of education and to treatment in the "least restrictive environment" appropriate to their needs. This support has been instrumental in facilitating the return of institutional persons to the community and in preventing the placement of others into institutions.

Federal government departments have supported the process of deinstitutionalization by linking financial assistance to state governments with various requirements and standards. One significant incentive to deinstitutionalize was that federal funding for placement of persons into nursing homes and other facilities was more favorable than that for retention in institutions.

Admissions to institutions and waiting lists have been drastically reduced and eliminated in some states. However, many disabled persons still enter, re-enter, or remain in institutions when they could be served adequately in the community. The number of persons in publicly supported institutions for the mentally retarded actually increased from 176,500 in 1963 to 193,200 in 1967, but declined to 181,000 by 1971, and to 168,300 (a 7.5% reduction) between 1971 and 1975 (this last estimate was made by the National Association of Coordinators of State Programs for the Mentally Retarded). The reduction would appear to correlate with the extensive use of nursing homes and intermediate care facilities in lieu of institutional placement. Some of these "alternate" facilities are so large that, in effect, persons move from one institution to another.

Not only has the institutional situation not changed as it should have, in relation to the increased availability of human and fiscal resources, but with the higher and more demanding expectations generated by normalization and equal rights concepts, local community services are under-performing.

One reason for the under-performance of local community services is the tradition of specialized, segregated community programs and facilities, making integration and public attitude change difficult to accomplish. Another contributing factor is that responsibility for local community service is generally fragmented and unclear. In spite of a dramatic increase in the number of community services and facilities available, substantial shortages remain, and those that are established are often poorly coordinated and not optimally utilized. The ability to link and coordinate services is often impeded by the confusion over program entitlements and the categorical nature of funding.

A salient problem at all levels of government is that the agencies with primary responsibility do not have, or control, the funds

necessary to develop comprehensive community-based care systems in demand by the advocates of the disabled population. They
are not granted sufficient funds or responsibilities for regulating
or monitoring the standards of care within the community services and facilities. In order to implement comprehensive service
systems at state, regional, and local levels, a unified national
strategy or management system is needed.

Although various offices, task forces, and committees, as well
as the Developmental Disabilities Act of 1970, were designed to
assist the states in providing and coordinating an array of programs and services, the mechanisms needed to coordinate the
plethora of efforts by the many federal departments and programs impacting on the field do not exist at present.

Within the past decade numerous programs have been implemented to realize and overcome the problems involved in the
development of state and regional coordinated service delivery
approaches. Under President Jimmy Carter, action has been initi-
ated to consolidate a variety of subdivisions within HEW, involving such bodies as the Office of Human Development, Rehabilitation Service Administration, Developmental Disabilities Office,
and the President's Committee on Mental Retardation.

## Canada

The population of Canada (23 million) is approximately one-tenth
that of the United States. Although larger in land area, the settled
and most densely populated areas are concentrated along the
United States-Canadian border. Both countries function with similar local, state, or provincial and federal geopolitical systems.
Although both national governments provide approximately half
the funds to the state or provincial governments for cost of human
services, United States federal agencies are generally more influ-
ential in determining program direction, particularly with respect
to mental retardation. Division of power and responsibilities for
human services between levels of government in the two countries
is dissimilar. In the United States educational field, the federal
government has a distinct and direct role, whereas the Canadian
counterpart does not. The Canadian government shares costs in
higher education, health, and welfare, but the provinces tend to
have more program self-determination in the provision and coordination of services for the disabled. A greater local dependency
for program development and activity has been created by the

United States government, because of its massive grant programs, its large central technical-professional program planning
establishment, and its overall complexity of public and private national bodies concerned with mental retardation.

In contrast, the Canadian Association for the Mentally Retarded (the equivalent of the National Association for Retarded
Citizens in the U.S.) is the only major nongovernmental advocacy
body in Canada. There are no mental retardation divisions per se
within the federal system, such as the President's Committee on
Mental Retardation in the United States. The Canadian Association for the Mentally Retarded (CAMR) is a federation of 10 provincial and 380 local organizations with approximately 30,000 members. In contrast, the National Association for Retarded Citizens
(NARC), with 50 states and 1,800 local units, has about 150,000
members. The Canadian volunteer movement would, therefore,
appear to have a more concentrated citizen-action movement relative to population (roughly 10% that of the United States).

The CAMR serves as the major link between the professional-
technical interests and the citizen movement, assuming a very
significant role in influencing specific nationwide program directions. With increased complexity of the system came the problem
of the effectiveness of the citizen movement. In 1963, the Canadian Association decided that changes must be instituted if the
citizen movement was going to continue giving ongoing, effective
leadership.

In the face of such growing complexity and technology, it was
felt that citizen power effectiveness was dependent upon the support of good technical power. In response, the Canadian Association developed, and currently operates, the National Institute on
Mental Retardation (NIMR) as a means of linking the citizenry with
program technology.

A major impetus for the securing of national consumer
strength in Canada is that the federal government is only indirectly involved in the administration of human services (except
employment). Education is the complete responsibility of provincial education departments. There is sharing of costs with the federal government for social services, vocational rehabilitation, and
supplemental income. Also, Canadian law has made it virtually
impossible for citizens to launch class-action suits against government. Thus, consumer power remains the most viable tool for ac-
complishing change. Voluntary nonprofit organizations can function in a quasi-partnership fashion with governments at the na-

tional level. There are also relatively few proprietary (private-for-profit) operations, which further enhances the role of the nonprofit organization.

Political pressure in Canada for improving the conditions and services for its mentally retarded citizens may be somewhat less intense than in the United States. Canadian health and social services have developed along universal coverage lines with less categorization. The federal agencies have tended to discourage categorical programs. In general, therefore, the service program structure, generic and special, is much less complex than those "south of the border."

Although there are well established differences in the structure for the development and provision of services in the two countries, the quality and level of (comprehensive) programming for handicapped persons are quite comparable at this time. One comparative measure relates to the status of institutional residency and placement in both countries. Canada had an institutionalized resident population of approximately 19,172 in 1971, and 18,950 in 1976. This parallels the situation in the United States. Since the general Canadian population increased by over 1 million (to 23 million) between 1971 and 1974, the proportionate institutional population decrease is even more significant. This decrease is probably due, in part, to the same contributing factors alluded to in the United States. Disabled persons were shifted to community services, but some of these moved from residency in older overcrowded "Hospital Schools" to new or remodeled smaller institutions—now renamed Regional Resource Centres.

In Canada there is not the same fiscal incentive from federal authorities to reduce institutional populations as is witnessed in the United States. Consequently, Canada has not resorted as much to the use of intermediate care facilities, which are generally not staffed or prepared for this role, in order to reduce institutional populations in compliance with federal incentives. The community living alternatives in Canada have been largely in the hands of the nonprofit sector with government funding, as opposed to the use of proprietary boarding and nursing homes. This arrangement has reduced incentive for "dumping." Placement in community facilities is more likely to be delayed until the availability of good quality and appropriate alternate services exists.

Over the past 8 years there has been a remarkable growth in the number of group homes and community facilities that serve as acceptable alternatives to institutional placement. Yet the continuing demand for institution admissions and readmissions, along with the slowness of the decline in Canada's institutionalized populations, suggests that the presently existing community services are as yet an uncertain alternative.

## THE NEED FOR A GUIDING IDEOLOGY

Ideology is to human services operations what the profit motive is to business enterprises. It provides the incentive to improve and to create better solutions. As the threat of conflict, including war, stimulates technological progress, so an ideological thrust provides management with new tools with which to realize higher level goals.

An effect of the "equal rights" and "normalization" precepts for handicapped individuals has been to motivate ever larger numbers of people to view human services problems from new and different approaches. Examples are seen in the establishment of "least restrictive alternative" and "range of options" (or "choices") concepts in the planning and development of residential, vocational, and other opportunities; the greater use of generic agencies as a step toward more "integration"; assistance to families for early (home) stimulation of the child; Parent-to-Parent and Citizen Advocacy schema; evaluation methods, such as PASS (1), the use of legislation and litigation to obtain and apply the rights of disabled persons; and the development of Comprehensive Community Service Systems (2).

## BARRIERS TO CHANGE

In countries or areas with extensively developed services the obstacles to progress relate not so much to the lack of ideology as to the difficulty in achieving the transition. The ideology tends to be accepted but present systems are in a period of turmoil, in which the new ideology and philosophy have not been sufficiently tested and demonstrated to have created sufficient public pressure to help those who are coping with immediate crises to make the transition in program implementation.

The ultimate adverse effect of past growth patterns is a gradual buildup of external and internal impediments to future progress and change. The special and segregated facilities and programs developed to date, such as schools, workshops, and Special Olympics programs, are highly visible (and relatively permanent) and therefore serve as effective public image codifiers. They clearly indicate to the public that authorities on the subject (namely, the parents, professionals, and others who do the planning and managing of buildings and programs) would appear to believe in segregation as the best solution, thus creating and entrenching a public perception that segregation is needed rather than modifying it. Another problem that develops is that the investments by service clubs, associations, and governments that have gone into (segregated) buildings and programs are so extensive that they seem to feel obligated to be protective and often defensive about them. All these factors impose external impediments to change.

Certain internal impediments to change develop as well. There is security in shutting out the "normal" world—a security found in isolated kinds of programming. Special segregated programs also often tend to resist integration with normal services because the originators (including parents) of the service come to believe that others are not as capable or as accepting and/or would discriminate against the disadvantaged if placed in a normal environment. Also, a sense of "ownership" frequently develops. Parents inherently do not want to move their offsprings from the setting in which they are settled, even when the situation is less than reasonable or ideal.

Reactions to new concepts are generally passive or moderate as long as the new ideology, with its implied criticism of existing activity, has insignificant support or limited publicity. Radical concepts like integration of minority groups encounter or generate resistance in direct proportion to the perceived threat they pose to the status quo.

By 1966, the Council for Exceptional Children (CEC) had grown into a significant professional body on the premise that education for the handicapped had to be special and segregated. It came as a mild shock when, that year, its president challenged the validity of that concept. However, the real resistance developed when the concepts were presented in the form of proposals to school boards. It then became a double-edged sword, threatening first the special education field itself and, second, the regular teaching field, which had been relieved of the responsibility of coping with disabled children.

There often is at least short-term validity to much of the resistance to change to new concepts that have not been tested or probed. It would be less than responsible for parents to turn against the complete protective environment of large residential or segregated educational and vocational facilities in hope that local community service systems could provide an equivalent generic alternative since the latter have as yet not generally proved themselves in that regard.

A more insidious reaction to new ideologies is to feign adaptation to changing concepts. This can be done by modifying definitions or making self-interpretations of terms and concepts to create merely a cosmetic change. Thus institutions are re-labeled "resource" or "developmental" centers; meetings to discuss common problems (with no follow-through) are portrayed as evidence of coordination; the word "comprehensive" is used to describe partial range of services; professionals working in relative isolation next to each other in rehabilitation settings refer to their effort as "interdisciplinary," when, in fact, a more precise description would be "multidisciplinary"; "citizen advocacy" becomes a new word for established social casework techniques; and "individual program plans" (IPPS) and "general service plans" (GSPS) are new terms for "case conferencing" and "team approach."

In other words, some apparent modification occurs, but fundamental change is avoided. A well-established and effective political technique is for more conservative minded parties or governments to take the ideas of radical-minded ones and introduce them under another designation in a modified "incremental" fashion. This may occasionally represent a superior approach to realizing improvements, but it can also have tragic consequences. Some governments have closed down or reduced the population of large residential facilities by transferring the residents to private nursing homes (also known as intermediate care facilities) without necessarily changing or easing the problem. Ironically, this is done in the name of "normalization" and "integration." Such practices could often be better described as "dumping" than "integration."

## SYSTEMIC APPROACH TO PROBLEM SOLVING

A systemic organizational methodology is a necessity for major progress in the field of mental retardation. The underutilization of existing knowledge and methodology account for the present limitations of real progress in the attainment of current delivery service goals.

The knowledge and experience exist for futuristic planning with a high degree of predictability. Given, for example, certain data about the nature and direction of an organization, the rise and decline of a democratic organization can be predicted with relative reliability by those knowledgeable and experienced in the field of organizational dynamics, as can the probable success or decline of a particular human service organization. Thus realization of significant change in human services requires the establishment and support of (nondirect service) operations or entities whose sole function is to gather and analyze data, evolve and promote new concepts and test them (through experimentation and demonstration) on a limited scale basis before attempting universal application. Such activity or operations must be given reasonable freedom of action, generous support, opportunity to experiment, and the challenge to prove the practicality of new concepts. The agencies for change must be competent; have a broad base of support; have a creative, energetic, and committed work force; and an adequate, clear-cut time frame in which to work.

For success we need: a) a clear objective of the goal and the motivation and determination to do what is required for success, b) an appreciation of the potential contribution of the basic and applied sciences and an understanding of the diverse elements that need to be coordinated and focused, and c) a catalytic vehicle capable of mobilizing and integrating the technical knowledge and resources with the socio-political (decision making) forces.

In Canada, the citizen movement representing the field— CAMR—undertook to develop such a catalytic entity through the establishment of the NIMR. The NIMR was designed as a problem-solving entity that would stimulate the translation of existing knowledge into action plans. More specifically, the need for NIMR's development was seen as follows: a) The practitioner and scientist lacked adequate ways of effectively communicating with each other; could an entity be created that could facilitate this? b) Positive changes in attitudes toward research, training, and service program activities, and toward retarded people themselves, are best stimulated by dynamic, well-informed, and organized citizen action groups. How could these be supported in such efforts? c) Flexible characteristics of dynamic radical volunteer movements are prone to give way to the more typical rigidity and defensiveness associated with any group that develops vested interests once initial goals have been achieved. Could an institute help revitalize such movements? d) It was assumed that, in order for a citizen movement to maintain effective leadership and remain a catalyst for change, it needed to develop a technical-professional sophistication of its own in parallel with governments, institutions of higher learning, professional groups, and other agencies.

Establishing a workable plan that could bridge the technical professional elements with a citizen action movement required an innovative organizational approach in which the technical and nontechnical interests would need to mutually participate and share. The plan for such an entity was conceived in 1963, but the NIMR formally began operations in 1970. The Institute is owned and operated by the CAMR and located on York University Campus, Toronto. The facility has training and research facilities, and serves as the nation's major technical and professional resource for governments, institutions of learning, and agencies serving the disabled. A major asset is the National Library and Reference Service, consisting of general and technical information—the most complete documentation center in the country. Programs include manpower utilization and training, research and evaluation, program development, legislation, consumer organization revitalization, and international developments. The objective of the NIMR is to function as a major catalyst for influencing and accelerating major change on a national scale. Realizing greater utilization of existing resources requires a monumental and complex plan of action involving extensive research into modern organizational systems. There are needs for the development of plans and guidelines, large numbers of specially trained personnel (staff and volunteers), evaluation systems, and improved governance models; necessary also are strategies to change attitudes toward newer program philosophies and concepts, innovative service program delivery approaches, and methods to overcome resistance to change from workers in the field, governments, and public and the voluntary movement itself.

The Institute is viewed by the volunteer members of the CAMR as having a unique and special status unlike a conventional national office. The Institute's effectiveness is increased by being able to relate directly to governments and agencies that more readily accept services from a technical institute than from a national office of a citizen action movement.

Since the evidence to date suggests that technical institute operations under the direction of citizen movements accelerate and reinforce the voluntary organization itself, this could become a significant pattern in other countries in the coming decade. There is a potential to realize a network of national and international institutes for a worldwide exchange of technical and service data, techniques, and personnel, representing the critically important component in overcoming the barriers to applying and utilizing existing knowledge. (The 26 Caribbean nations' Caribbean Association for Mental Retardation has developed a Caribbean Institute on Mental Retardation modeled on the NIMR, and Australia is developing similar plans.)

## MODEL COMMUNITY SERVICE SYSTEM NEEDED

The challenge of this decade, in the area of developmental disabilities, is to develop a plan that could realize rational, effective, and cost-beneficial human service delivery systems, capable of providing a wide range of service options. After extensive study, the NIMR proposed a long-term national goal for Canada for a more advanced service delivery system than currently exists. In September, 1971, CAMR adopted a goal for the development of comprehensive community services for the developmentally handicapped across Canada as its "Plan for the 1970s." This project, referred to as ComServ (Comprehensive Community Service Systems), is a model program plan designed to narrow the gap between knowledge and practice, taking top priority in the concerns and interests of CAMR and NIMR.

Fundamental to the ComServ plan of directives is a regional (regions within states or provinces) approach to service delivery. The advantage of a regionalized service system over a local service system is that it permits greater specializations of services, counters excessive provincialism, provides greater cost efficiency through small experimental scale models, allows better utilization of expertise, and has a greater impact on other agencies and governments. The advantages over provincial or state services is that the regional system fosters closer client-family ties, has a greater sensitivity to local conditions and needs, and increases the identification of citizens with services. ComServ's success depends heavily upon the involvement and action of the citizen or consumer movement.

It is an ambitious long-range plan that requires supreme effort, extensive financial and human resources, and coordination between the consumer organization and technical-professional resources. The role of NIMR is to bridge the gap between theory and practice, enabling program specialists and others to bring their respective powers to bear on either local problems or national issues affecting the disabled population. This model is based on a premise that there may already be sufficient funds expended and that resources exist to meet the needs of the disabled population, but that fragmentation, duplication, lack of coordination, and maladaptation of resources contribute to an illusion of shortages. ComServ is designed to provide mechanisms for overcoming the problem of central and local government's inability to establish the necessary coordination for a comprehensive service delivery system.

The variety and quantity of services included in a comprehensive system (a ComServ model) are much greater than previously anticipated. Basic service requirements fall into five groups or subsystems of the total service system.

## Family Resource Service Subsystem

The family resource service subsystem consists of a range of services (or choices) to enable disabled persons to remain in the community with their own families or in adoptive, foster, or group homes. It consists of such services as genetic counseling and testing, assessment and diagnosis, individual and family counseling, information resources, lending libraries, financial subsidy, crisis assistance and respite care, visiting homemakers, in-home parent/child training, and transportation. The challenge is to ensure that every family will receive the type and amount of service necessary to maintain the disabled individual in the family or a substitute local community environment.

## Child Development Subsystem

The child development subsystem includes developmental programs for preschool age children, elementary through secondary public school education, and post-school programs. Special units or programs must be available to provide behavior shaping in the case of hyperactivity, distraction, extreme withdrawal, or other major behavior problems. Physiotherapy, speech therapy, and other highly specialized services are made available to multiply handicapped and severely retarded children in need of such services—ideally provided by existing community-based children's services.

## Vocational Services Subsystem

The vocational services subsystem calls for a spectrum of vocational choices and supports to meet the specific needs of each individual, challenging each individual to move to higher levels of independence and productivity. Vocational options include sheltered work in industry, on-the-job training, work situations in commerce and industry (such as work stations), trades training and employment, self-employment, and other options still to be identified.

## Residential Services Subsystem

The residential services subsystem emphasizes a range of residential opportunities concerned with where disabled persons live and what is provided in addition to receiving shelter. Home living options are given first priority. The second priority is the establishment of housing options that closely approximate the home. The third group of residential options is designed to meet special needs, providing the needed back-up that allows the other, less restrictive, options to remain flexible. These options require some trained staff and full supervision.

## Protective Services Subsystem

The protective services subsystem is a range of activities and programs coming into existence that service planners are learning to combine and modify so that they can protect people and property in their community living situation. Protective services should include legal guardianship, property management, trusteeship and representative payee, protective service workers paid to track and follow up handicapped persons, corporate advocates, free legal aid, and representation and citizen advocacy.

ComServ requires a sound organizational and sound administrative structure. In addition to the subsystems described, a central services subsystem is called for to hold the system together and increase efficiency and effectiveness. The distinguishing components are administration (senior staff), fiscal control, staff development, evaluation, research, and public education.

In the envisioned design, central (state or provincial) government has responsibility for establishing global policies, priorities, and implementive strategies, and in addition certain general regulations and standards for services, which are established and enforced within the sub-areas or regions. Central government retains the power but service delivery is delegated to the structure closer to the people requiring the services.

The chief function of regional service system directorate is to see that needed services are provided and coordinated in the region by conducting long-term planning for comprehensive services on a regional basis. The directorate also determines regional policies and strategies as well as local priorities. Development of local funding sources and allocation of funds and the employment of direct staff to carry out these functions are additional responsibilities.

Regional bodies need to be responsible for control of direct administration of services and for funds made available from central government. They must have the right to purchase client services, have authority for service agency coordination, and obtain funds besides those granted by the central government. Regional bodies working on a purely voluntary basis (without real authority) are unable to develop and manage an effective and coordinated comprehensive system.

The ComServ process must be introduced gradually because of the impossibility of reorienting all existing services at the same time. The Institute proposed establishment of a limited number of experimental and demonstration (E&D) projects that will test and develop ComServ's method of organizing and delivering community services in the various regions. NIMR recommended that there be no more than one suitable area in each of several Canadian provinces selected as an E&D region.

To assure the quality and success of the E&D ComServ projects, 12 criteria were developed for selecting and approving any project before it is accepted. There are six criteria for regional suitability: 1) sufficient population size to justify a wide range of services, 2) accessibility of a region to transportation routes, 3) availability of professional resources, such as institutions of higher learning, 4) community receptivity to the project plan, 5) strong consumer and related organizations inside the region, and 6) prospects of local and long-term funding sources. Another six criteria for program suitability include: 1) a plan to offer a wide range of service options, 2) evidence of strong project direction, 3) commitment to the demonstration role, 4) applicability of the demonstration lesson to other regions, 5) willingness of regional personnel to accept consultation, and 6) the adoption of some specific research missions.

## MANPOWER NEEDS

Critical to the success of the ComServ model is the development of knowledgeable and able leadership and a supportive attitude base. There is an extreme shortage of staff and volunteers trained and experienced in organizational systems approaches and modern change agentry in the field of developmental disabilities.

The Institute analyzed personnel needs and evolved what has become known as a "national manpower model." The "model" has a basic premise that many of the jobs presently performed by professionals can be performed as well by less highly trained front line volunteers and staff. Some three-quarters of the work force does not require university level training. These people can be trained in community colleges in 1- or 2-year programs. Better supervisory and leadership skills should be provided to the others who are trained in higher education programs. This calls for alterations in present university programs to develop in their graduates the essential leadership skills.

The manpower model proposes a four-level system of training and recognition of personnel in the field. An important part of the hierarchy is that workers have clear routes and opportunities for moving up the ladder, as well as having their functions and status within the system clearly defined.

The Level I staff members are basic care workers performing in a technician capacity. They can aspire to a higher level by obtaining the required additional educational training and practical experience. At Level II the individuals are being trained for some leadership abilities. Level III is equivalent to the bachelor's degree person trained at universities with some specialization. The Level IV category of workers includes those in management and administrative capacities and the various professional disciplines (3).

## CONCLUSION

The systems knowledge, methods, and resources for establishing a comprehensive spectrum of services and the manpower necessary for its implementation are potentially available. With continued consumer competence in systems organizations and the continuation of parent-professional partnership movement, the legacy of institutionalization for handicapped persons can become past history, as adequate community living programs are realized.

## QUESTIONS AND ANSWERS

QUESTION: What do you perceive as the most important role of NIMR?

ROEHER: I conceive its primary role as a stimulator for influencing and accelerating major change in service program development—toward improved program quality and providing the range of service options (choices) that the handicapped person is entitled to, to act as a citizen with equal rights and opportunities for self-realization of his or her potential. Moreover, it serves as a bridge between the technical-professional and the consumer elements in the field.

QUESTION: What has been happening in terms of ComServ's training developments for the Level III and IV workers?

ROEHER: The NIMR has undertaken short-term upgrading courses for Level III and IV workers (or those with University level training in the field of human services). This is an interim measure because of the shortage of advanced training opportunities in Canada at the university level.

QUESTION: Do you detect untapped opportunities for cooperation between Canadian and American programs?

ROEHER: Yes. Variations of experimental or innovative programs like ComServ are being launched in both countries and, although there is some collaboration, more needs to be done to share experiences and pool resources.

QUESTION: What single development do you feel is most necessary for progress in the next 5 years?

ROEHER: The launching of more experimental and demonstration ComServ-type projects in both countries and interchange of findings. ComServ calls for empowered coordination of community resources and this accounts for present resistance to launch even experimental programs of this nature. It is the only true alternative to institutions but it requires interagency team work beyond the typical voluntary coordination.

QUESTION: Are we missing any opportunities to influence broad public attitude change toward developmental services?

ROEHER: Yes. The public requires evidence that the generic and specialized community agencies have the interest and commitment to coordinate their resources to serve the handicapped in the same way that the normal population is provided for.

The public's view and attitudes are based on what the service agencies do. If they use segregated approaches to serving the handicapped, the public will believe that is what is best, and vice versa.

There was a time when the blame could be placed on the public. The situation is now reversed. Enough money is being spent to serve the needs of the handicapped, but too much of it is low yield due to agency performance.

## REFERENCES

1.  Wolfensberger, W., and Glenn, L. 1975. Program Analysis of Service Systems. National Institute on Mental Retardation, Toronto.
2.  Comprehensive Community Service Systems. The Plan and guidelines for the development of ComServ programs are available from the National Institute on Mental Retardation, York University Campus, Toronto, Canada.
3.  The National Manpower Model. National Institute on Mental Retardation, Toronto.

# KEY ISSUES
# AND CHALLENGES
# BEFORE US

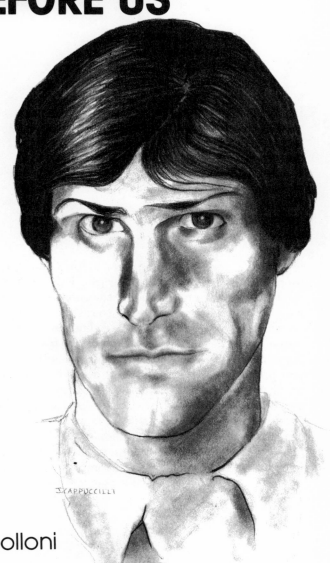

J.CAPPUCCILLI

Tony Apolloni

*The chapters of this book present a kaleido-*scope of opportunities and concerns. This summary chapter is intended to underscore some of the most salient issues and challenges facing us as we attempt to reshape residential services for citizens with special developmental needs. In identifying common elements in the recommendations made by the authors of preceding chapters, I focus attention on some of the central conceptual and pragmatic factors affecting deinstitutionalization and community development efforts. The movement to develop high quality, community-based residential services is in its infancy. The chapters on Michigan, Nebraska, Pennsylvania, and Canada share the wisdom of service pioneers. Other chapters share the perspective of family members, advocates, and researchers. This final chapter represents my attempt to abstract and spotlight what appear to be cornerstone considerations for successful community systems.

## NORMALIZATION

The premier program systems described in this book share a common commitment to the principle of normalization (1, 2). This similarity may be a vital ingredient in each system's success. Citizens achieve most when they coordinate efforts to achieve commonly held societal goals. Coordinated, cooperative actions are facilitated by adherence to a shared value system. The principle of normalization provides a rallying point for a truly inspired human service movement, a movement that holds promise for energizing service planners, providers, and consumers. Normalization involves a process—the application of culturally typical teaching strategies— and a product—culturally acceptable appearance and behavior.

Widespread confusion exists regarding the meaning of normalized services. The concept is too often defined through citing a litany of common abuses. In the ultimate sense, normalization means doing everything possible to accentuate people's positive attributes while striving equally hard to diminish their negatively valued characteristics. Normalized programming entails securing needed prosthetic devices, supplying powerful teaching technologies, structuring rewards for staff and clients to motivate personal growth, and allowing persons with special needs to reside, learn, work, and enjoy themselves in the same settings as all other persons. Normalized programming also entails avoiding the segregation of persons in institutions; prohibiting large community-based residences (those with four or more clients); eliminating segregated, duplicative social and medical services; and avoiding the juxtaposition of socially devalued groups (as when elderly or minority workers are exclusively recruited as human service workers).

Normalization holds two mandates for society. First, ordinary citizens must expand their tolerance of and acceptance for people who are different. Second, social services must be instituted that allow all persons the opportunity to *be an individual person and to be treated like all other persons to the maximum extent possible,* i.e., to be independent of the supervision of others, to be productive, and to contribute to society.

Once social planners, service delivery agents, and consumers commit themselves to ensuring normal life-styles for developmentally atypical individuals, needed actions become clarified. Normalization stands like a lighthouse as a referent for human service activities. It promises to revolutionize our perception of services for people who are different. It redefines the role of service providers from that of "taking care" of people to doing whatever is culturally appropriate to help people grow to the maximum extent possible. People are no longer viewed as representatives of a disability category. They are viewed as *individuals with disabilities* and as handicapped only to the extent that society allows their disabilities to block mainstream social participation.

Systemic commitment to normalization clarifies the role of caregivers. Normalization principles provide the theoretical basis for making consistent everyday decisions. I have found the following questions useful to evaluate the accord of caregiver behavior with the principles of normalization:

1.  Are my activities promoting the full physical and social integration of the persons I am trying to assist?
2.  Are my activities accentuating their positive characteristics and life opportunities?
3.  Are my activities diminishing the harmful effects of their socially devalued features and personal misfortune?
4.  Are my activities incorporating the full benefits of prosthetics and modern teaching technology?
5.  Are my activities facilitating realistic consumer self-control and productivity versus promoting consumer dependence on other-controlled environments?

## STAFF TRAINING

The quality of care and supervision afforded to consumers by human service workers is likely proportional to the care and support supplied to workers. Consistent with the recommendations expressed earlier in this volume, service systems should:

1.  Develop a policy statement on staff training in the area of residential services
2.  Make licensing and vendorization of residential services contingent upon training
3.  Make mandatory training available for personnel at all levels throughout their career
4.  Offer incentive pay to staff when they attend training and provide subsidies to consumer organizations that provide training

5. Employ existing service providers as trainers
6. Make training competency based and continuously evaluated

## ADVOCACY

As reviewed by Al Zonca, several types of advocacy are important to ensure adequate services for disabled citizens. First, assistance is called for in the area of person-to-person friendship. Many individual needs may be met through small but intimate amounts of sharing between advocates and protégés. The citizen advocacy movement has great potential for combating the negative influences of the materialism and competitiveness that characterize United States social order. Training in consumer self-advocacy, both for primary consumers (service recipients) and secondary consumers (family, guardians, and conservators), is crucial. We must always keep in mind that the emergence of services for our constituency has been motivated by consumer, largely parental, pressure on government. The Canadian Institute on Mental Retardation outlined by Allan Roeher is a promising model of how consumers may effectively tap theoretical and technical sophistication to shape valid social services.

Legal advocacy is also of crucial importance. Persons with special needs have the same entitlements as all other members of society, plus other rights, such as to treatment, that are unique to labeled populations. The past decade has witnessed an unprecedented acceleration in society's attempts to provide fair and equal treatment to disabled persons. These attempts are largely attributable to legislation and litigation ensuring open access to community living. Constant vigilance is demanded, however, to ensure that economic pressures and special interest groups, such as those described by Pieper and Cappuccilli, do not erode recently won advances.

Systemic advocacy also seems vital to developing humane and nonstigmatizing social services. Coordinated, comprehensive systems are called for to provide continua of residential, educational, and vocational services that meet the needs of individual consumers. Integral feedback mechanisms are necessary to supply data on the cost of services per increment of client growth and on the relative life-style qualities afforded by various programmatic alternatives. Protection and advocacy bodies, independent of fiscal reliance on government, are needed to guard against the abridgment of consumers' natural and legal rights by powerful bureaucratic systems. Information networks are called for that facilitate a continuous flow of information regarding advocacy efforts. Existing advocacy efforts must receive added support and new advocacy concepts and mechanisms must be developed.

## NONSTIGMATIZING LANGUAGE

History is replete with instances of institutionalized discrimination and socially dehumanizing practices aimed at devalued social subgroups (3). Inhumane treatment is clearly facilitated through stigmatizing or stereotyping subgroups with pejorative terms. The labels and professional jargon surrounding persons with special developmental needs provide an excellent illustration of this phenomenon. Many of the labels for this group, such as the "mentally retarded" or "mentally defective," obscure the myriad normal human and developmental characteristics exhibited by citizens with special developmental needs and set apart the people so designated. Whenever one social group successfully rationalizes the nonhumanness of others, tragic results follow. Recent attempts to legalize the removal of life support systems for brain injured infants provide a dramatic illustration of the inhumanity that may be directed toward persons labeled deviant (4).

New terminology is needed within human services. This language must not stigmatize, dehumanize, or stereotype the members of our constituency, but rather it must give full recognition to their humanity and to our brotherhood. The beginnings of such language change are currently emerging. Persons with disabilities are termed "persons with special developmental needs" to verbalize acceptance for individual differences in developmental pace and course. Moreover, concepts like "handicappism" (5) are focusing attention on those who profit by applying clinically useless terms to others. The terms used in reference to consumers by most of the authors in this volume appear to reflect awareness of this problem. We must tap the collective creativity of consumers and professionals to accelerate the trend away from degrading terminology. Eventually, perhaps, we will be successful in displacing the language of disability and exceptionality with a language of growth, ability, and humanity.

## DEVELOPMENTAL MODEL

The developmental model should be embraced by the total human services community because it asserts a positive view of client potentiality and an empirically substantiated position relevant to program conduct and organization (6). It recognizes that human beings thrive only to the extent that they are allowed to change and develop. Notions of fixed and stable characteristics long dominated the thinking of professional disciplines. The developmental model holds that human characteristics are in a constant state of change due to interactions between individual behavior and environment and that the course and pace of human development may be altered and enhanced by intentional arrangements of prosthetic environments. If we are to truly embrace the developmental model, we must not only realize that our constituency is composed of people capable of astounding developmental progress, but that service providers must work in a rigorous, intentional, and accountable fashion to design and evaluate environments that assist consumers in actualizing their full developmental potential.

The developmental model has direct implication for the design and organization of human services. Maximally effective human service programs must rely on the best of current instructional technology and must be delivered in concert with a continuum of program alternatives. Programs must be technologically sound and coordinated in a developmentally relevant fashion if clients are to persistently progress toward independence and productivity. Instructional systems are now appearing that provide step-by-step plans for expanding consumers' developmental progress (7, 8).

## SCIENCE AND TECHNOLOGY

We must stimulate communication between the scientific and service-providing communities. Professional associations like the American Association on Mental Deficiency and the Council for Exceptional Children have demonstrated abiding commitments to scientific research on the nature, causes, prevention, and treatment of handicapping conditions. Too often, however, the results of these efforts have had little impact on the lives of consumers. Emphasis should be placed on translating both basic and applied research findings into language that is useful to community organizers, practitioners, and consumers.

New technologies, capable of great positive impact, may be derived from sound research. The widely lauded California Project offers an excellent prototype (9). This project has disseminated a teaching technology, based on sound experimental research, that provides guidelines for efficaciously teaching vocational and developmental skills to persons with special developmental needs. Here the continuum of science to teaching technology to widespread social significance is in evidence. Systematic replications are badly needed in many additional areas of programming.

## RESIDENTIAL SERVICE CONTINUA

We must continue to develop and support personal living arrangement continua to allow persons with special developmental needs access to homelike, community-based services in their own homes and/or communities. Bronston's chapter sketches many of the fundamental features important to such services. Skeletons of needed systems currently exist in many states, including numerous islands of community programming excellence like those described in the chapters by Provencal, Hitzing, Knowlton, and Roeher. Future developers should attend closely to the lessons available from these more developed systems. The following considerations seem particularly important:

1.  Emphasize the adoption and implementation of the principle of normalization. Shared commitment to ideology is essential to effective service development.
2.  Avoid the establishment of permanent, facility-based services that inhibit flexible programming. Services must change over time in response to shifts in client characteristics and societal opportunities.
3.  Design and deliver services on an individualized basis. Begin by assessing the client's needs, not the available placement options.
4.  Begin by developing the most integrated elements of a service continuum and initiate specialized or segregated services only when absolutely necessary. Support generic services with resources and hold them accountable toward the needs of our constituency.
5.  Stress quality control and monitoring from the onset of service delivery. Feedback is essential regarding the rate of clients' development, the quality of life they experience, and the cost of services.
6.  Accept that it takes time, i.e., years, to establish service continua for broad geographical areas. Learn to be persistent but patient.

7. Emphasize staff development. Recognize that the care received by clients is greatly affected by the care we exhibit in training service providers. Staff training should be mandatory, criterion referenced, ongoing forever, and clearly linked to a career development program.

8. Involve consumers in planning and evaluating services. The genesis of human service development in this country rests on the efforts of parents committed to helping their disabled children. Parents are an essential political ally to comprehensive service development.

9. Promote expansion of coordination among state and local agencies to curtail fragmentation, gaps, and duplications in services. Projections of reduced resources to support human services make interagency cooperation a necessity.

10. Ensure a reciprocal relationship between the amount of protection (i.e., care and supervision) provided in a setting and the amount of guidance or training it supplies. Highly protective settings should also provide intense levels of developmental training so that clients may learn to live more independently.

## SUPPORT SERVICES

We must develop networks of community support services. Establishing a viable community system entails more than providing community residences. We must also act to modify the unavailability of meaningful education and employment opportunities, inaccessible transportation systems, nonexistent medical and dental services, and the unavailability of assistance in consumers' adjustments to recreational and social experiences. Consumers must be educated to rely on generic versus specialized resources whenever possible, e.g., churches, movie theaters, bowling centers.

It is important that integrated support services be established if living in the community is to truly affect consumers' lives. For example, educational services that are segregated do not afford appropriate peer models, do not provide a normal referent to shape teacher expectations, do not permit consumers to regularize their behavior in relation to real-world pressures, and do not allow nondisabled children opportunities to benefit from the developmental diversity exhibited by children with special needs. It is up to us to design service models that permit the full physical and, to the maximum extent possible, social integration of persons considered disabled. As Jerry Provencal has noted, it is an easy and obvious excuse to avoid fully integrated services because we fear that the public will not accept our constituency. Instead, we must accept responsibility for achieving a highly ambitious reformation in social tolerance. We must increase our expectations of ourselves and of our fellow men and engineer to achieve success.

## DEINSTITUTIONALIZATION

Increased community placement has become a political, economic, and legal necessity. Health systems across the country are changing, not just improving. Improvements in behavioral technology, revisions in human service ideology, legislative and court mandates, accreditation standards, and decreases in human services budgets are forcing reductions in the number of persons residing in large state institutions. Institutions are said to provide inadequate role models, set limits on client growth, result in whole groups of clients being treated similar to the most dependent member of their group, render consumers unable to make choices, and are characterized by insufficient staff at the direct level of care, drug abuse, and excessive costs. Unfortunately, the available community alternatives frequently offer even poorer care. Community services in most areas are either nonexistent or may be characterized as possessing inadequate rate structures, underpaid and untrained staffs, insufficient support services, and poor monitoring and accountability. Community placements are sometimes merely institutions that serve fewer clients. As in large state institutions, clients eat, sleep, and participate in recreational activities in a single setting.

The program systems described in this book offer living examples of comprehensive, community-based models. Their long-term stability and systematic replication are essential. The major factors delaying deinstitutionalization in California, as in the rest of the United States, are: 1) organized opposition from hospital employees, 2) organized opposition from the parents of hospitalized clients, and 3) the underdevelopment of community services. The fact that the recent suit to depopulate Pennhurst State Hospital was filed by the parents of hospitalized consumers illustrates the importance of the third factor. The Pennhurst parents saw a viable community system (see Mel Knowlton's chapter) and wanted their children out of the hospital and into community services.

Parents and mental health employees want service continuity and permanence and, in most places, both see the hospitals as the "tried and true" route to attaining these goals. We must address these concerns by developing model community services that provide service and employment security. My personal interactions with parents and hospital personnel suggest that many would prefer community settings, given equivalent services and job security.

## BROAD-SCALE PUBLIC SUPPORT

Public relations efforts are called for to make ordinary citizens aware of the human rights and economic issues involved in establishing comprehensive, community-based services. We must take our message to the ordinary citizen. A recent review of attitude-change films in the area of developmental services, carried out by Joanna Cappuccilli, revealed that most films are either ideologically sound but of poor technical quality or ideologically unsound and of good technical quality. New media are needed, addressed to general audiences, that portray the aspirations we hold for our constituency's future. We must illustrate the essential commonality in the behavior and needs of all people—disabled and nondisabled alike. We must learn to effectively use the public media—television, radio, newspapers, and magazines.

## CONSTITUENCY EXPANSION

We must broaden the base of our constituency to include all persons who exhibit similar, special developmental needs; elderly persons, temporarily disabled individuals (one of every seven citizens), physically disabled persons, persons labeled "mentally ill," and those with sensory impairments and other disabling health conditions. These special interest groups share many functional characteristics and could profit from similar social services in areas like transportation, attendant care, housing, and employment. Bureaucratic structures that set up competition between these groups are problematic. If we work together we are much more likely to succeed. We must learn to appreciate the common cause of all socially devalued persons. The nature of personal needs must take precedence over the etiology of the condition underlying the need.

## TOGETHERNESS

The primary purpose of this volume and of the conference that generated it is to build awareness of alternatives to traditional residential treatment approaches being applied with persons labeled "developmentally disabled." The authors are service system pioneers and consumer advocates. Their message in one respect seems crystal clear: "Once service providers 'stand with the victims' of America's human service system and demand compliance with consumers' rights to effective treatment and habilitation, the service system will begin to change." Alternatives must be recognized and developed. Planners and providers must be flexible and perceive that today's needed services may be obsolete next year. Cooperation, trust, mutual respect, open sharing, and accountability are essential among planners, providers, and consumers if a successful human service movement is to emerge.

## REFERENCES

1. Wolfensberger, W. 1972. The Principle of Normalization in Human Services. National Institute on Mental Retardation, Toronto.
2. Way To Go. 1978. University Park Press, Baltimore.
3. Farber, B. 1968. Mental Retardation: Its Social Context and Social Consequences. Houghton Mifflin Co., Boston.
4. Florida State Legislature. 1972. Sunshine Bill.
5. Biklen, D., and Bogdan, R. 1975. Handicappism. Human Policy Press, Syracuse.
6. Bijou, S., and Baer, D. 1965. Child Development. Appleton-Century-Crofts, New York.
7. Westaway, A., and Apolloni, T. (Eds.). 1978. Becoming Independent: A Living Skills System. Edmark Associates, Bellevue, Wash.
8. Adams, P., Apolloni, T., Cooke, T. P., Palyo, B., Raver, S., and Sabbag, D. (Eds.). 1978. Sonoma Developmental Curriculum. Human Services Associates, Santa Rosa, Cal.
9. Galloway, C., and Lecours, R. G. 1978. Try Another Way in California. Mark Gold & Associates, Urbana, Ill.

# Index